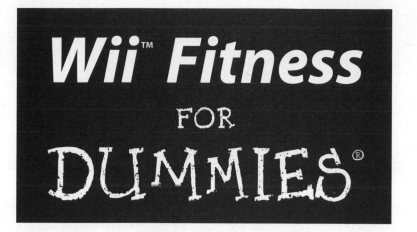

Wii™ Fitness
FOR
DUMMIES®

by **Christina T. Loguidice**
Bill Loguidice
American Fitness Training of Athletics (AFTA)
Certified Personal Trainers

WILEY

Wiley Publishing, Inc.

Wii™ Fitness For Dummies®

Published by
Wiley Publishing, Inc.
111 River Street
Hoboken, NJ 07030-5774
www.wiley.com

WILEY

About the Authors

Christina T. Loguidice holds a Bachelor's degree in English and German from Rutgers University and has made a name for herself in scientific, technical, and medical (STM) publishing, beginning her career at Springer-Verlag in production. Since that time, Christina has gone on to oversee several peer-reviewed medical journals, including *Surgical Rounds, Resident & Staff Physician,* and *Cardiology Review.* She is currently the editor of *Oncology Net Guide* and *OncNurse.*

In addition to her background in STM publishing and being well-versed in the latest cutting-edge medical research, Christina is an American Fitness Training of Athletics (AFTA) Certified Personal Trainer and a Black Belt in Tae Kwon Do. She has been a fitness enthusiast for more than 10 years.

Bill Loguidice has a Bachelor's degree in Communications from Rider University. Bill has been a longtime business, technology, staffing, and creative professional. He has contributed to various business, entertainment, and medical periodicals, including *U.S. 1, Video Game Collector,* and *Surgical Rounds,* writing and developing ideas on a broad range of topics. A videogame and personal computer collector since before it was trendy, Bill is presently the cofounder and managing director for the online publication Armchair Arcade, one of *PC Magazine*'s Top 100 Websites for 2005. Bill is also the cofounder of Myth Core, a creative development company.

As a top videogame and computer historian and collector, Bill personally owns and maintains more than 350 different systems from the 1970s to the present day, including a large volume of associated software, accessories, and literature. It is from these great resources and his passion for the topic that Bill is often called upon to provide subject matter expertise to both public and private media interests, including the *Las Vegas Review-Journal* and the *Orlando Sentinel.* He is also coauthor of the book *Vintage Games: An Insider Look at the History of Grand Theft Auto, Super Mario and the Most Influential Videogames of All Time* and a writer and producer for an upcoming feature-film videogame documentary from Lux Digital Pictures.

In addition to his impressive credentials in technology, Bill is an American Fitness Training of Athletics (AFTA) Certified Personal Trainer. He has been a dedicated fitness enthusiast for more than 20 years and is uniquely positioned to combine the benefits of a healthy lifestyle with videogames.

Dedication

Christina Torster Loguidice: I dedicate this book to my husband, Bill. Few people get to work on a project of this scope with their best friend, and I truly feel blessed to have this opportunity. I also dedicate this book to our girls, Amelie and Olivia, who fill our lives with unimaginable love and ensure that there is never a dull moment. Finally, I dedicate this book to my parents, Ulla and Wolfgang, and my sister, Brigitta, who have always believed in me and been my cheerleaders.

Bill Loguidice: I would like to dedicate this book to my family, including my amazing wife, Christina, my beautiful daughters, Amelie and Olivia, and of course my parents, Jody and Bill, and sister, Alicia, whose enthusiastic support for my work is always appreciated.

Authors' Acknowledgments

We'd like to thank the great team at Wiley for their support on this project, particularly our direct contacts, Beth Taylor and Amy Fandrei. We'd also like to give special thanks to Didi Cardoso of Gamer's Intuition for the technical review. Last, but certainly not least, we'd like to thank our literary agent, Matt Wagner, for helping us land this project in the first place.

Publisher's Acknowledgments

We're proud of this book; please send us your comments at http://dummies.custhelp.com. For other comments, please contact our Customer Care Department within the U.S. at 877-762-2974, outside the U.S. at 317-572-3993, or fax 317-572-4002.

Some of the people who helped bring this book to market include the following:

Acquisitions and Editorial

Project Editor: Beth Taylor

Acquisitions Editor: Amy Fandrei

Copy Editor: Beth Taylor

Technical Editor: Didi Cardoso

Editorial Manager: Jodi Jensen

Editorial Assistant: Amanda Graham

Sr. Editorial Assistant: Cherie Case

Cartoons: Rich Tennant
(www.the5thwave.com)

Composition Services

Project Coordinator: Lynsey Stanford

Layout and Graphics: Melissa K. Jester, Christin Swinford, Christine Williams

Proofreader: Debbye Butler

Indexer: BIM Indexing & Proofreading Services

Publishing and Editorial for Technology Dummies

  Richard Swadley, Vice President and Executive Group Publisher

  Andy Cummings, Vice President and Publisher

  Mary Bednarek, Executive Acquisitions Director

  Mary C. Corder, Editorial Director

Publishing for Consumer Dummies

  Diane Graves Steele, Vice President and Publisher

Composition Services

  Debbie Stailey, Director of Composition Services

Table of Contents

Part II: EA Sports Active: Personal Trainer 121

Introduction

*E*xercise and gaming — who thought the twain would ever meet? At least not until *Wii Fit* came along. Sure, there were other fitness titles on other platforms prior to the Wii, but Nintendo's console really helped bring the genre mainstream. Why is this? Well, for the first time, there was a way to accurately track even subtle body movements and provide feedback in real time. *Wii Fit* was engaging, giving you the sense that a personal trainer was right there with you, and you weren't just haphazardly mimicking actions observed onscreen while a lifeless automaton cycled through the same repertoire of encouragement.

Certainly, as with all things, there are skeptics. Some may even smirk upon seeing a "videogame" book categorized as a fitness title, but those folks likely never gave "exergaming" a try or are hardcore fitness enthusiasts who spend hours pumping iron or putting the treadmill to its paces at the gym. There is certainly nothing wrong with that, unless taken to the extreme, but even if we wanted to, most of us simply don't have the time or resources to devote to that type of lifestyle. For us, exergames can be a great and fun way to make regular physical activity a part of our lifestyle, rain or shine.

We concede that some fitness titles are certainly better than others at yielding results and offering guidance and feedback, but we believe if you try any of the games covered in this *For Dummies* book—*Wii Fit Plus, EA Sports Active: Personal Trainer, Jillian Michaels Fitness Ultimatum 2010* — you will feel like you are doing your body good (be sure to turn to Chapter 14 to get a glimpse of even more games). Time is exceptionally precious in this harried world, and our goal is to help you make the most of the time you devote to these Wii fitness titles.

Conventions Used in This Book

Our objective is to help you get away from some of your conventions of daily living — those things that you do day in and day out — by helping you incorporate Wii fitness in your life. To facilitate this, we use *conventions* throughout this book. Although it seems ironic using conventions to get away from conventions, consistency is important when it comes to writing, especially when the objective is to provide an instructional guide.

To lead you on your Wii fitness journey, we always refer to exercises the way that the manufacturer does, even if its title seems a little off. For instance, we cover *Tricep Extension* and *Jumping Jack* in Chapters 3 and 11, respectively, even though these are more commonly referred to as *Triceps Extensions* and *Jumping Jacks*. This allows you to easily identify the exercises covered in the software in this book.

Whenever any of the equipment is mentioned, such as the Balance Board, Wii Remote, Leg Strap, and Resistance Band, these items are captialized. This allows you to more readily identify any necessary equipment when skimming sections of the book.

We also use the word click quite a bit throughout, such as click the A button or click the Next button. The Wii Remote functions much like a computer mouse and the word *click* best describes the required action. Last, whenever we provide you with URLs for Websites, these appear in monospace font, ensuring they stand out. After all, these URLs are important to help you troubleshoot any issues with your equipment or to expand on the software's offering, allowing you to boost your Wii fitness potential.

Why You Need This Book

In discussing *Wii Fitness For Dummies* with family, friends, and other individuals, some questioned, "Do you really need a book for that?" If you are reading this section, you are no doubt wondering this yourself. After all, these games generally have easy-to-navigate interfaces and do a great job of guiding you through each activity by demonstrating movements and providing feedback, making a *For Dummies* book seem superfluous. Although this book does provide you with a reinforcement of what the games already do well, its scope goes well beyond that.

Contained within these lovingly crafted pages, you also find tips on optimally performing the activities and navigating menus, suggestions for alternatives or variations on the exercises, additional routines, and countless useful figures and tables for quick reference. We also delve into exercise theory and physiology, dispelling common myths and noting how these activities can benefit your body. Most of the activities offered in each of the titles we cover, namely *Wii Fit Plus, EA Sports Active: Personal Trainer, and Jillian Michaels Fitness Ultimatum 2010,* are common exercises. Our goal is to give you a solid understanding of how to perform these activities so that you are confident in your ability to perform the exercises even without the guidance of your Wii.

How to Use This Book

Unlike works of fiction or other narratives, this book does not have to be read in a linear fashion or in totality for that matter. Each section stands alone, and some parts may be more useful to you than others because this book covers three distinct fitness titles, some of which you may not own. Identifying the parts that are most relevant to you is a breeze thanks to the *For Dummies* style. Each chapter contains many subsections, each of which is outlined in the book's comprehensive table of contents, and every chapter features an "In This Chapter" introduction, which includes a bulleted list of the chapter's scope. With this setup, you are never left wondering what's covered. If you still can't find what you're looking for, turn to the index, where you can search for a topic alphabetically instead.

As for more specific uses, if you have just purchased one of the titles covered in this book, consider going through the part of the book devoted to that title before popping the program into your console. If you don't have time to read that entire section, at least glance at the Getting Started chapter for that program, which will give you a good sense of what to expect from the game and allow you to make the most of the program from the very beginning. For example, when playing *EA Sports Active: Personal Trainer,* you may be tempted to use a Guest Pass the first time you play, but if you read Chapter 7, you find out why it makes sense to establish a fitness profile from the get-go.

You can also use this book to get a quick overview of an exercise. Although you will want to watch any tutorial videos before performing an activity for the first time, you may not want to watch them subsequently. You can use this book to get a quick overview of an activity before performing it; for instance, if you forgot an arm or foot placement.

Finally, having three fitness titles outlined in one book allows you to easily compare activities and capabilities between the different games. This can be handy if you own multiple titles, as it can facilitate deciding which game you want to work out with at any given time. It can also help you decide whether to purchase one of the games you don't yet own. So dig in, digest, and enjoy.

Foolish Assumptions

Whether your exercise bike is collecting dust or you are already a fitness enthusiast, we assume that you bought this book because you are looking to incorporate Wii fitness in your life. Our goal is to help you achieve this, no matter how much or how little guidance you need. For Wii or exercise novices, there is support throughout this book on navigating the software and performing the exercises. On the other hand, for those more experienced in either area, there are countless tips, scoring and gameplay information, exercise variations, and other fitness and Wii tidbits that may help enhance the Wii fitness experience.

Although some of the activities in the book do not require a Wii Balance Board, and many of the activities in each of the three software titles covered here — *Wii Fit Plus*, *EA Sports Active: Personal Trainer*, and *Jillian Michaels Fitness Ultimatum 2010* — could be performed even without a Wii, we assume you either own a Balance Board or are looking to invest in one, as it greatly expands your Wii fitness options.

How This Book Is Organized

This book is divided into four parts; the first three cover a popular fitness title for the Wii. The fourth is the Part of Tens, a staple of *For Dummies* books; it provides an overview of fitness accessories and other exercise titles available for the Wii. Each part consists of several chapters, all of which have multiple subsections. To find the information you need, you can simply skim chapters, refer to the table of contents, or peruse the index. Of course for maximum benefit, you can also read chapters in their entirety, which we hope you will.

Part I: Wii Fit Plus

Part I consists of six chapters. Chapter 1 provides you with an overview of *Wii Fit Plus,* including everything you need to know to get started, such as familiarizing yourself with the Balance Board and navigating the menus. Chapter 2 details the series of body tests that you will be asked to perform to establish a baseline and monitor your fitness progress. The remainder cover each exercise category offered by *Wii Fit Plus,* including yoga, balance games, strength training, and aerobics.

Part II: EA Sports Active: Personal Trainer

Part II, which starts with Chapter 7, gives you the information you need to get started. It examines the equipment that comes with this title, including the Resistance Band and the Leg Strap, and covers how to navigate the menu, establish your fitness profile, use the fitness journal, and more. Chapter 8 covers the available exercises, which are broken out by upper body, lower body, cardio, and sports activities. The last chapter covers the routines, from selecting preset to customizing your own; we even give you a few specialized routines that you can try.

Part III: Jillian Michaels Fitness Ultimatum 2010

Some may wonder why we decided to include this title in the book, especially since its predecessor, *Jillian Michaels Fitness Ultimatum 2009,* received rather poor reviews overall. Certainly this game is not of the same caliber as *Wii Fit Plus* or *EA Sports Active: Personal Trainer,* but it offers a unique approach to working out with its less traditional exercises and more ballistic activities, such as swing kicks and water pump. Part III starts with an overview of this title, including navigating the menus, creating your character, enrolling in the Hell-week style boot camp, and tracking your stats. The second chapter in this section reviews the training options and discusses how to determine your regimen based on your objectives. The final chapter provides an overview of all the exercises.

Part IV: The Part of Tens

Part IV includes two chapters. The first, Chapter 13, gives an overview of the fitness and other accessories that you may want to consider to enhance your workouts, covering everything from exercise mats to wireless Nunchuks. Chapter 14 offers a glimpse of ten other fitness titles for the Wii that you may want to consider adding to your Wii fitness library.

Icons Used in This Book

In the left-hand margins of this book, you notice one or more icons, each of which has a distinct purpose and is vying for your attention. The three icons used are as follows:

As the name implies, this icon draws attention to information that you can make use of. It generally involves an action item, such as how to perform an activity or an alternate technique you can consider.

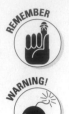

This icon signifies tidbits we want you to keep in mind. Some of this stuff you may already know, but because there is no way to tell, repeat we must. Besides, isn't repetition one of the keys to memory?

This icon signifies cautionary items. It highlights an action that can result in injury or an unintended consequence when making certain menu selections.

Where to Go from Here

We hope you go home with this book and absorb it all, but in all seriousness, where you go from here is entirely up to you. You can read it cover to cover or take a look at the table of contents, index, or just flip through the book to find areas that interest you.

Regardless of where you go, we hope that this book will serve as a useful guide in helping you achieve your fitness goals. If we've neglected to cover something or you have any questions or comments you'd like to make, we'd love to hear from you. Feel free to e-mail us at `wiifitness@ armchairarcade.com`.

Thank you for reading.

Part I
Wii Fit Plus

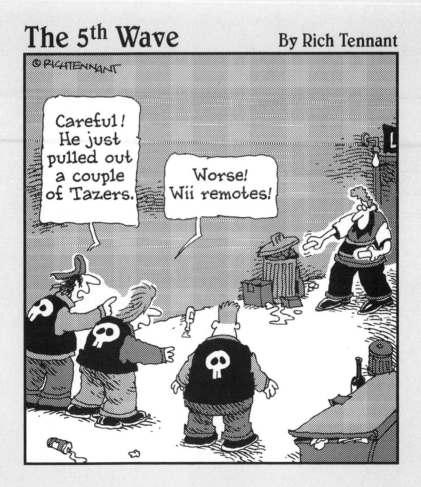

In this part . . .

Welcome to a life of improved health and well-being with Wii fitness! This part of the book details Nintendo's insanely popular *Wii Fit Plus* and many of the core exercise concepts that translate to the other Wii fitness games and working out in general. Here you are introduced to the *Wii Fit Plus* software and the revolutionary Balance Board accessory. You also learn about your center of balance, body mass index, and the other important health information gleaned from *Wii Fit Plus*'s various fitness tests. Next, you dig into the yoga and strength training exercises, and then proceed to the section on My Fit Plus, where you gain important knowledge about calories, exercise routines, and more. Then, you learn how to get your heart pumping by jumping into aerobics. This section concludes with an overview of the Training Plus and balance games, which are both fun and challenging.

Chapter 1

Getting Started

• •

• •

After you make the decision to incorporate *Wii Fit Plus* into your healthy lifestyle, the first step is to set up the system. Unlike most games, setting up *Wii Fit Plus* is a multistep process befitting its unique combination of sophisticated hardware and software. This chapter helps to make this process a breeze so that you can get down to the serious — yet surprisingly fun — business of working out.

In this chapter, you find out how to set up *Wii Fit Plus* to work with your Wii console. You also discover how to activate your Balance Board, prepare your Mii for the activities ahead, and establish your baseline physical fitness level. We go over what the Balance Board can and can't do, how the Wii Remote and Nunchuk are used, and how to navigate around the many *Wii Fit Plus* menus.

Introducing Wii Fit Plus

One of the major reasons the Wii Fit phenomena has been so strong is because it relies on a unique bundled peripheral called the Balance Board. This innovative wireless controller has become the face of the Wii fitness revolution, adding a new dimension of interactivity far beyond what is possible with just the Wii Remote and Nunchuk.

Although the original Wii Fit features over 40 strength training, aerobics, yoga, and balance activities, the exercise experience is unstructured and mostly solitary. Although not a radical change, *Wii Fit Plus* adds over 20 more activities, provides preset routines and customizable workouts, has a

Metabolic Equivalent of Task (MET) calculator that tracks calories burned based on how much exertion is required to perform a movement, and offers far more robust multiplayer support, making this updated version a worthwhile investment for old and new Wii fitness enthusiasts alike.

What's in the Box

Wii Fit Plus comes in two flavors: a box set with the *Wii Fit Plus* software and the Balance Board, or, for those who already own the original Wii Fit, just the *Wii Fit Plus* software.

Inside the oversized *Wii Fit Plus* box, shown in Figure 1-1, you find the following:

- **Wii Balance Board:** The plastic Balance Board is a flat, rounded, rectangular platform that can support a standing weight of up to 330 pounds. Through four Balance Sensors located on the bottom of the board, both weight (pressure) and balance can be measured. The board is battery operated and communicates wirelessly with the Wii console via Bluetooth, just like your Wii Remote.

- ***Wii Fit Plus* software:** Like most other Wii software, the *Wii Fit Plus* program comes in a plastic snap case that contains the *Wii Fit Plus* game disc, instruction booklet, registration information, and marketing material.

- **Wii Balance Board foot extensions:** If you plan to use the Balance Board on a thick carpet, one extension can be placed on each of the four balance sensors to provide sufficient clearance under the bottom of the platform to ensure proper measurements.

- **Wii Balance Board Operations Manual:** An instruction manual specific to the Balance Board hardware. A portion of this information is repeated in the *Wii Fit Plus* instruction booklet.

- **AA batteries:** For the Wii Balance Board to function, the four included batteries or suitable replacements must be placed in the well under the battery cover on the bottom of the board. Quality AA batteries can last approximately 60 hours.

Carefully remove these items from the box and discard the packing materials properly. You may wish to save the *Wii Fit Plus* box for future storage or transportation of the Balance Board, particularly because it features a convenient carrying handle.

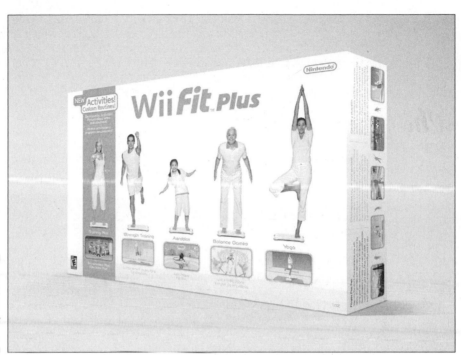

Figure 1-1:
The front
of the full
Wii Fit Plus
bundle.

Hooking Up the Components

At this point we assume you already have your Nintendo Wii set up and working, and at least one Mii stored on your console. If not, refer to the Wii Operations Manual that came with your console or, for additional detail, *Wii For Dummies* by Kyle Orland (Wiley Publishing). As for *Wii Fit Plus,* follow these setup steps after inserting your disc and starting the game, and you can be on your way to fitness and fun in no time flat:

1. **Press A on your Wii Remote after you are comfortable with the Wii Remote Strap Usage screen instructions or simply wait to automatically proceed.**

   If this is your first time playing *Wii Fit Plus,* you will have to create and save data and synchronize the Balance Board.

2. **On the *Wii Fit Plus* save-data creation screen, press A on the Wii Remote.**

If you are upgrading from Wii Fit, *Wii Fit Plus* makes use of your previous data. After the save data has been created, a confirmation screen appears. Press A again. If you already have Wii Fit data, you are taken on a brief tour of *Wii Fit Plus*'s new features, and you can either skip ahead to the "Incorporating the Wii Remote and Nunchuk" section of this chapter, if you want a refresher on controller functionality, or go straight to the "Navigating the *Wii Fit Plus* Menus" section. Otherwise, you'll be prompted to sync the Balance Board to the Wii.

3. **Remove the battery cover on the bottom of the Balance Board and insert the four AA batteries if you have not done so already. Then press the small red SYNC. button, as shown in Figure 1-2.**

   The blue power light on the Balance Board should now be flashing.

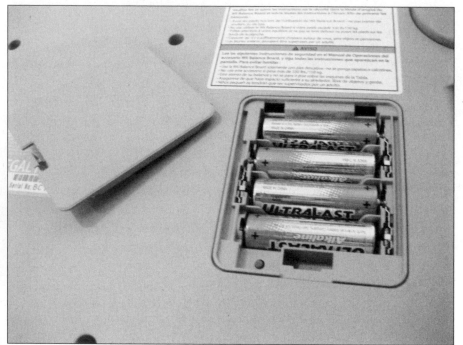

Figure 1-2:
The Balance Board with the battery cover removed.

4. **Open the SD Card slot cover on the front of the Wii console next to the system disc slot. While the blue power light on the Balance Board is still flashing, press the red SYNC. button on the Wii console, as shown in Figure 1-3.**

   The power light on the Balance Board stops blinking and remains lit after the synchronization is complete.

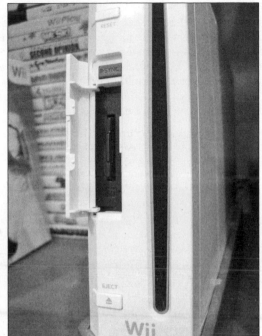

Figure 1-3:
The open
SD Card slot
cover on the
front of the
Wii console.

Do not press and hold the rectangular SYNC. button on the Wii console for more than ten seconds; otherwise, all synchronization information for all your Wii Remotes will be deleted and you'll need to resynchronize them per the instructions in the Wii Operations Manual.

5. **Close the SD Card slot and Balance Board battery cover. Return the Balance Board to its upright position.**

Only one Balance Board can be registered to a single Wii console at any one time. Any new Balance Board synchronization will overwrite the current registration information. Because the Balance Board uses the Player 4 connection, any board-compatible software is limited to a maximum of a single board and three other controllers.

If all steps were followed correctly, the virtual Wii Balance Board greets you and serves as your animated anthropomorphic tour guide when you're playing *Wii Fit Plus*.

After a brief intro, you are asked to verify your console's date and time. If the settings are correct, use your remote to select Correct; otherwise choose Incorrect and make the necessary adjustments.

You are asked to choose a Mii already saved on your Wii system to represent yourself. The Miis from the Mii Channel's Mii Plaza appear on your screen in groups of up to ten. If you have more than ten Miis on your system, you can click the arrows on the left and right sides of the screen to scroll through the list or press – or +, respectively, on your Wii Remote. Select your favorite virtual representation of you and press A on your Wii Remote to confirm.

Establishing Your Baseline

Now that you've confirmed the date and time and chosen the Mii for you, the virtual Wii Balance Board begins to step you through the introductions, which you can choose to read or skip. The first major task the virtual Wii Balance Board will have you do is a quick Body Test to establish your physical fitness baseline, which includes your weight, Center of Balance, Body Mass Index (BMI), body control, and Wii Fit Age. Turn to Chapter 2 for a comprehensive explanation of each of these measures and the tests used to assess them.

Initial body measurements

When prompted, enter your height and birth date. Point and click on either the up or down arrow on the screen to increase or decrease the values, respectively. After this information is entered, you are prompted to either change or accept the data by pressing OK. After you're satisfied, click OK.

Be sure to enter your real birth date for accurate analysis. If for some reason you're concerned that others who will be playing your *Wii Fit Plus* will be able to see this or your other personal information — such as your weight — you have the opportunity to enter a personal identification number (PIN), described later in this chapter, so only you have access to these data.

Follow these steps to create your baseline readings:

1. **Place your Balance Board directly in front of the screen, three to ten feet back.**

   The board's power button should be facing away from the television, where the text for both Wii and Power on the top surface of the board is readable. After a brief synchronization, you are instructed to step on the Balance Board (be sure you're holding the Wii Remote).

   Before stepping on the Balance Board, ensure that there is sufficient clearance underneath, particularly if it is placed on a rug. If there is not sufficient clearance, use the Wii Balance Board Foot Extensions.

2. **Step on and remain still.**

   If you move, or fidget, *Wii Fit Plus* will have trouble taking a baseline reading and you'll be instructed to step off and restart the process. After *Wii Fit Plus* gets a successful reading, it will ask how heavy your clothes are: Light (-2 lbs.), Heavy (-4 lbs.), or Other. Use your best judgment and select your answer using the Wii Remote and pressing A. If you select Other, you can press up and down on your Wii Remote's directional pad to respectively raise or lower the starting value of 0 lbs.

   It is recommended that you use the Balance Board barefoot. Socks can be too slippery and shoes might not provide enough range of motion or the tactile response necessary to perform certain activities. One good alternative to bare feet is to wear non-slip Yoga, Pilates, or "toe" socks, which provide traction and a full range of motion with minimal tactile loss.

   After you step on the Balance Board, a large green semicircle starts moving on the screen. This represents your Center of Balance. Try to keep the green semicircle centered.

   Wii Fit Plus now prompts to measure your Center of Balance. If you fidget too much, you have to start over, so it is important to have a relaxed, stable stance. If you remain sufficiently still, you receive your Center of Balance results. Don't worry if your balance is dramatically off center, as this is just an initial reading, and as you continue to use your *Wii Fit Plus,* your results should improve.

3. **When ready, continue pressing the A button to proceed through the informational prompts until you come to the first test.**

   You are now asked to align your Center of Balance by shifting your bodyweight until the red dot rests in the blue circle in the middle of the onscreen Balance Board.

4. **After you receive your results, press the A button to proceed.**

   You should now see your Body Mass Index, or BMI, results, which is a rough measure of body fat based on your height and weight. You will learn more about BMI in Chapter 2, but for now just accept the verdict as an arbitrary baseline that will be useful as a future point of reference to improve upon.

   Don't be alarmed if *Wii Fit Plus* changes the appearance of your Mii's waistline in either direction. Remember, *Wii Fit Plus* can't see how you really look; it can only guess based on statistics, which don't always reflect reality.

5. **Press A to show two menu options, Weight and Next.**

   Selecting Weight shows how much you weigh in pounds. If you select your weight, you have the option of going back to the BMI screen or clicking Next. If Next is selected, you are taken to the Body Control tests.

The Balance Board is said to be more accurate than the average bathroom scale, so if you find your weight to be completely off, it could be because you don't have enough clearance below your Balance Board, indicating foot extensions are warranted. See "Understanding Balance Board Capabilities" later in this chapter for more on this. Some variation in weight is normal, however, and your weight can fluctuate by several pounds each day.

Body control baseline

Because this is your first time using *Wii Fit Plus,* your body control assessment starts with the Basic Balance Test. For a more comprehensive overview of this test, turn to Chapter 2.

To set up your body control baseline, follow these steps:

1. **Press A on the controller until you reach the Basic Balance Test, where you are presented with brief instructions and a prompt to press A to start. Spread your feet evenly apart on the Balance Board and press A when ready.**

2. **Balance left and right on the board to keep each of the red bars in its respective blue area for three seconds.**

   You go through a few practice rounds before the countdown to the real trial, which challenges you to make often dramatic left and right shifts and then hold your position for three seconds. You have 30 seconds to finish all five rounds. If you are unable to finish them within the allotted time, you are given a default score of 30 seconds. The less time you take to finish the Basic Balance Test, the better your score.

3. **Press A to proceed.**

   After receiving either good-natured ribbing or praise about your Basic Balance Test performance, you are presented with your Wii Fit Age. Much like BMI, consider your Wii Fit Age, which is described in greater detail in Chapter 2, an arbitrary baseline that will be useful as a future point of reference.

4. **Press A on the controller until you're prompted to stamp your progress on the calendar. Point your Wii Remote at your TV screen and press A to stamp today's date with a footprint.**

   Congratulations, you're now official!

5. **Press A to continue after reading each of the information prompts until you reach the Goal screen.**

   Wii Fit Plus suggests a goal based on your analysis. For example, if you're overweight, it may suggest setting a goal to help bring your BMI down. Regardless of its suggestion, the goal is yours to set.

You can point and click on either the up or down arrow on the screen to increase or decrease your weight goal, respectively, which in turn shows the effect on your BMI rating, up or down. Be sure to set a reasonable initial goal: no more than a few pounds to gain or lose, depending on your needs. After your selection is made, you'll be prompted for a deadline. The default is two weeks from today, which is the minimum span of time and a figure you may or may not be able to increase depending upon what goal you selected. For example, if you selected to lose only one pound, the maximum amount of time you can set to reach that goal is three months. Alternately, if you selected to lose two pounds, the maximum amount of time can be set to six months. As you change your deadline, the calculation shown for what you'll need to lose or gain every two weeks changes as well. After selected, you'll be prompted to either Change your goal or to click OK to proceed. We discuss setting goals in more detail in Chapter 2, so for now, click OK.

You can make a new goal and deadline every week, so don't worry too much about setting this initial goal. It's more important at this early stage to familiarize yourself with the software and exercises.

6. **Press A to continue after reading each of the information prompts until you reach the Password prompt screen.**

Selecting Yes allows you to protect your profile with a password if you wish to hide your weight and other data from others. Using a password is discussed in detail in Chapter 2. For now, either select No or Yes. If you select Yes, you are asked to enter a four-digit PIN for a password. When prompted, reenter the number to confirm. Press A to continue through the information prompts.

You should now be prompted with the option to register a family member or friend (this prompt does not apply if you already have all eight available slots filled). Selecting No brings you to the Calendar screen, while selecting Yes brings you to the Wii Fit Plaza. See "Navigating the *Wii Fit Plus* Menus" later in this chapter for an explanation of your options at each of these screens. But first, let's find out more about the Balance Board.

Understanding Balance Board Capabilities

Your Wii Balance Board is a stylishly designed and solidly built technological marvel. Through its four evenly placed Balance Sensors located underneath, the board is able to detect both the amount and relative location of the pressure applied to any of its quadrants. The board can then wirelessly transmit these data to your Wii console in real time, just like your Wii Remote.

With support for a standing weight of up to 330 pounds and an impact force of over 600 pounds, the board accommodates a fairly broad range of individual body types, abilities, and general usage.

For the Balance Board to do its job accurately, you need to ensure that the sensors have sufficient clearance underneath, particularly if your Balance Board is being used on a rug. If any surface is touching the bottom surface of your board, you need to use the Wii Balance Board Foot Extensions to gain additional height. Placing the extensions is a simple process. Just follow these steps:

1. **Turn the Balance Board over and ensure that each of the four sensors is free of any dirt or debris.**

2. **Push one foot extension straight into each of the four sensors.**

   Ensure each extension is pushed in all the way so there is no imbalance.

3. **Return the Balance Board to its original position and verify clearance.**

   If there is still insufficient clearance under your Balance Board after placing the extensions, you either need to find a way to clear any obstruction or move your Wii to another, more suitable location.

Although a range of typically silicon non-slip covers is widely available in stores, the Balance Board already has its own textured surface. This textured surface is located on each half of the top of the board in an approximately 5 x 9-inch area, where you would roughly place each foot. For this surface to do its job, you must be barefoot or use non-slip socks, which also maximizes your range of motion and feel for the board.

Be sure to keep the Balance Board dry during exercise. Sweat on the surface of the board can make for a potentially slippery — and dangerous — situation. Having a towel handy is a big help!

Even if you never use your Balance Board barefoot or share its use, at some point your board will need cleaning. Remember that even though it may not look it, your Balance Board is a sensitive electronic device that must be treated with care. To clean your board, follow these steps:

1. **Wipe your Balance Board with a soft lint-free towel to remove any loose dirt or debris.**

2. **Wipe the board with a disinfectant wipe or a lint-free towel sprayed with a disinfectant cleaner.**

   Never spray liquids of any type directly on the board.

3. **Dry your board with a clean, dry, lint-free towel.**

4. **Allow the board to dry completely before use.**

If control on your Wii Balance Board seems inconsistent or otherwise incorrect, the typical culprit is depleted batteries. As with most electronics, a fresh set of batteries can make all the difference. If performance continues to be erratic after putting in new batteries, you can choose Settings in the Wii Fit Plaza and select the Wii Balance Board Check, which verifies proper sensor function. If your Balance Board has malfunctioned, visit `www.support.nintendo.com` or call Nintendo's hotline at 1-800-255-3700 for assistance.

Incorporating the Wii Remote and Nunchuk

Although most of *Wii Fit Plus*'s more interesting functionality revolves around use of the Balance Board, you still use your Wii Remote to navigate the menus and begin exercises. As always, before using the Wii Remote, it is important to use the wrist strap and Wii Remote Jacket for maximum safety, particularly because you are likely to be breaking a sweat.

Though not necessary, wearing shorts or pants with pockets is helpful so you can safely place the Wii Remote in them when performing running exercises. You can also opt to use other alternatives, such as the *EA Sports Active: Personal Trainer* Leg Strap, which is described in Chapter 7. Otherwise, you can simply hold the Wii Remote in your hand.

Be sure to familiarize yourself with the Wii Remote Settings menu. This menu is accessible at any time by pressing the Home button on an active Wii Remote and then clicking the Wii Remote Settings panel on the bottom of the screen with the A button. To leave this menu, click the Close Wii Remote Settings panel at the bottom of the screen or push the Home button again.

From the Remote Settings menu, you can change the Volume, Rumble, and Connection settings, each of which functions as follows:

✔ **Volume:** By clicking on the onscreen + and – buttons or pressing the same buttons on the Wii Remote, you can respectively increase or decrease the sound coming from the Wii Remote's speakers. Note that this setting remains the way you set it and applies to all Wii Remotes that will be connected to your system.

You may find that for activities like the Free Run and Free Step Aerobic Exercises — both of which are explained in Chapter 5 — being able to adjust your Wii Remote's speaker volume is essential.

✔ **Rumble:** This option determines whether the Wii Remote vibrates to certain onscreen or in-game options. Unless you are sensitive to vibrations, it is recommended that you leave this option enabled for *Wii Fit Plus*. Like Volume, the Rumble settings remain and apply to all Wii Remotes that connect to your system.

✔ **Connection:** This option disconnects Wii Remotes from your console without turning off the system.

Unlike the Wii Remote, the Nunchuk attachment is used only for Rhythm Boxing, which is explained in Chapter 5, and Rhythm Kung Fu, Rhythm Parade, and Big Top Juggling, which are explained in Chapter 6. You are prompted by *Wii Fit Plus* when to use the Nunchuk. Because the standard Nunchuk is not wireless, it needs to be plugged in to the bottom of your active Wii Remote, after which it will be automatically detected. Like the Wii Remote, the Nunchuk can be used in either hand for maximum comfort.

Navigating the Wii Fit Plus Menus

Wii Fit Plus is divided into three main navigation areas: Wii Fit Plaza, the Calendar screen, and the Training menu. A fourth area, the *Wii Fit Plus* Channel, can optionally be added to the Wii Menu. The following sections explore the options available in these areas.

Wii Fit Plaza

The Wii Fit Plaza is the starting point for your *Wii Fit Plus* training. After all the Miis you registered in *Wii Fit Plus* have finished running in, you see the Wii Fit Plaza, as shown in Figure 1-4. The Wii Fit Plaza has the following options:

✔ **Wii Menu:** Click the Wii icon at the upper left of the screen to return to the Wii Menu screen. You can also return to the Wii Menu screen any time by clicking the Home button on your Wii Remote.

✔ **New Profile:** Click the happy-face, plus-sign icon at the middle left of the screen to create a new user profile. This new user has to go through the setup process we describe earlier in this chapter. After registration, the new Mii appears in the Wii Fit Plaza, ready to be selected.

✔ **Pet Stats:** Click the animal icon in the lower left of the screen to register User Data for your pet. You enter your pet's name, pet type (dog or cat), and characteristics. Although your pet will not be able to participate in the activities, your pet's weight can be measured and tracked. In addition, your pet's avatar appears during some of the activities to keep you company. Keep in mind that you can register only up to eight personal profiles, and this number includes your pets.

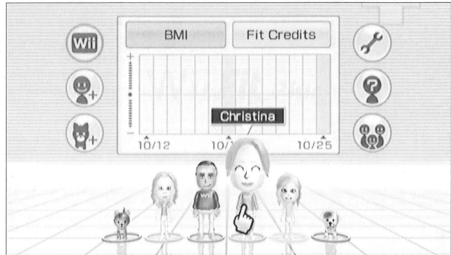

Figure 1-4:
The Wii
Fit Plaza,
showing a
highlighted
Mii.

Creating a profile for someone 3 years old or younger has the same restrictions as registering a pet. Once the baby is older than 3, all measurements and activities will become available. Keep in mind that whether you're holding a baby or pet, the Balance Board's 330-pound maximum weight limit still applies.

✔ **Settings:** Click the wrench icon at the upper right of the screen to bring up a submenu with the following options:

- **Install Channel:** This option installs the *Wii Fit Plus* Channel on your Wii Menu, which allows you to check your weight, BMI, and overall *Wii Fit Plus* stats without having to insert the *Wii Fit Plus* disc into your system. This Channel is described in greater detail toward the end of this chapter.

- **Wii Balance Board Check:** You can use this option to verify if the four sensors on your Balance Board are functioning. If every sensor has a check mark, your Balance Board is working as it should. If not, visit www.support.nintendo.com or call Nintendo's hotline at 1-800-255-3700 for assistance.

- **Credits:** Select the Wii Fit or *Wii Fit Plus* icon in the lower-right corner of the screen to see who helped make these titles possible. Pressing the B button at any time on your Wii Remote brings you back to the Settings menu.

✔ **Trial:** Clicking the question mark icon at the middle right of the screen starts up a trial version of *Wii Fit Plus,* which bypasses the standard Mii setup and registration procedure. After selecting one of six generic Miis, you can perform a basic Body Test or choose from a selection of 15 training games. Because this is just a trial, weight and training data are not saved, so this is most useful for giving your friends and family a quick demonstration of what *Wii Fit Plus* is all about.

✓ **Multiplayer:** Click the multiplayer icon in the lower right of the screen to access this mode, which allows you to use one or more of the Miis stored on your Wii console to participate in the nine multiplayer activities. Each player takes turns playing a single round and using the Wii Remote and Balance Board. Stats tracked in this mode are kept separate from those in the main *Wii Fit Plus* game.

✓ **Graph:** This large area centered in the top half of your screen displays the daily BMI measurements for all the Miis currently registered on your system unless their profiles are password protected. Select the Fit Credits button to change to the daily bar graph view of how much time you've been spending with *Wii Fit Plus* each day. You can isolate the data on a single Mii by hovering your Wii Remote over that player. You can also click anywhere on the graph and drag the Wii Remote pointer right or left to see earlier or later dates, respectively.

✓ **Miis:** Click on a Mii and then select Begin to Advance to the Calendar screen, which is discussed in the next section.

Calendar

The Calendar screen, as shown in Figure 1-5, is the first screen you encounter after registering a new Mii or choosing a Mii from the Wii Fit Plaza. The Calendar screen is also the secondary gateway to daily training with *Wii Fit Plus*.

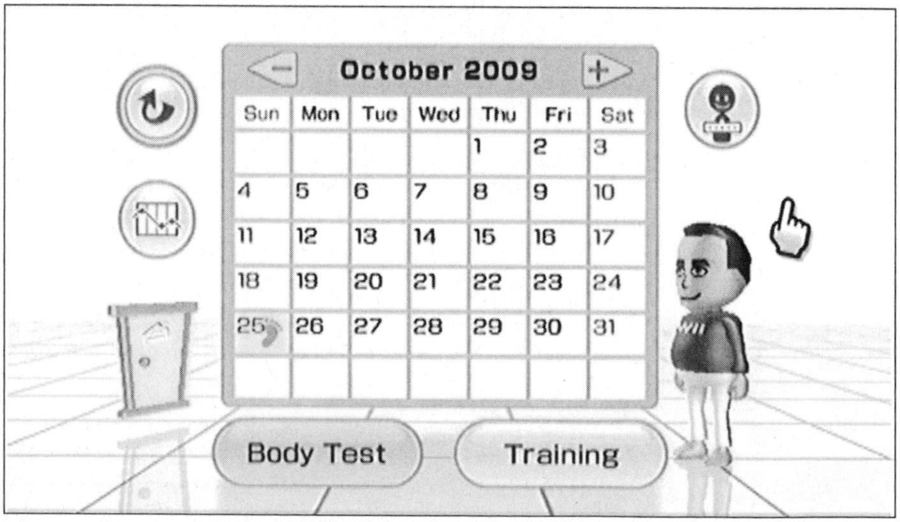

Figure 1-5: A sample Calendar screen. Every day you perform a Body Test, you get a stamp on your Calendar.

The options in this navigation area are as follows:

- ✔ **Wii Fit Plaza:** Clicking the return arrow icon at the upper left of the screen brings you back to the Wii Fit Plaza.

- ✔ **Graph:** Clicking the line graph icon at the lower left of the screen brings up a detailed chart of your Mii's daily progress. Use the buttons on the top row to toggle the graph's display between BMI, Weight, Wii Fit Age, Fit Credits, Waist, and Steps. Hover over a point on the graph with the Wii Remote to view a specific value for that day.

Waist and Steps measurements are entered manually. To measure your waist, bend at your side. The crease that forms indicates your natural waistline, which should be directly above your belly button and below your rib cage. Wrap a soft tape measure around your waist, directly on your skin. Exhale gently as you pull the tape so it remains taut against your body, but does not squeeze your skin. Your waist measurement is the number that meets the starting point of the tape. As for steps, you can measure these by using a pedometer. Some suggestions on what to look for in a pedometer are presented in Chapter 13.

You can click on the onscreen + and – buttons or press the same buttons on the Wii Remote to change the vertical and horizontal date range displayed on the graph. To scroll, click and drag the Wii Remote pointer anywhere on the graph. You can scroll farther by letting go of A and pressing it again. Click the Back button or press B on your Wii Remote to return to the Calendar screen.

- ✔ **My Wii Fit Plus:** A floating orange door appears in the lower left of your Calendar screen after the first time you access My Wii Fit Plus from the Training menu. This door is your instant portal to My Wii Fit Plus, saving you from having to take the long route via the Training menu to access this option.

- ✔ **User Settings:** Click the happy-face, word-balloon icon at the upper right of the screen to pull up a submenu with the following options:

  - • **Edit Profile:** Edit your Mii's height, date of birth, and password. Click an option, then use the onscreen arrows or + and – buttons on the Wii Remote to edit the information. Click OK when finished or press the B button on the Wii Remote to back out.

  - • **Change Design:** This option allows you to change your calendar color and choose a new design for your calendar stamp. The more you play *Wii Fit Plus,* the more stamps you unlock, up to a total of eight.

  - • **Save Time:** If you find that you consistently work out late at night and prefer your data recorded on a particular day, you can use this option to tell *Wii Fit Plus* to begin a new day at 3:00 a.m. instead of 12:00 a.m.

- **Delete User Data:** This ominous sounding option does exactly what it says, deletes all the stored data for your current Mii. If you choose Yes from the confirmation screen, all your measurements and hard work will be gone forever.

✔ **Calendar:** The calendar smack dab in the middle of the screen shows a stamp for every day you've performed a Body Test for the currently selected month. Click a stamped day to see the results of your BMI and Center of Balance tests for that particular day. Click the onscreen + and – buttons or press the same buttons on the Wii Remote to scroll through the months.

✔ **Body Test:** This option allows you to perform the Body Test for the day, as described earlier in this chapter. If you perform more than one Body Test in a day, the newest results will replace the previous results, provided you elect to save the more recent results. Because your body fluctuates throughout the day, you will often get different results. Try to do a Body Test only once each day and at roughly the same time each day for the most consistent results.

✔ **Training:** Opening this menu allows you to access the exercises you bought _Wii Fit Plus_ for in the first place. We cover this in the next section.

Training menu

If you're going to become fitter, you have to train for it, and that's where the aptly named Training menu comes in. The Training menu, shown in Figure 1-6, includes Training Plus, Yoga, Strength Training, Aerobics, Balance Games, and My Wii Fit Plus options. It is also where your Fit Bank resides, which we describe in greater detail a little later on.

Notice the virtual Balance Board in the background trying to get your attention? You can click on it to go to the Ultimate Balance Test or Scale Challenge, which are described in Chapter 2.

From the Training menu, click any of the options on the right-hand side to bring up the applicable training submenu. For information on Yoga and Strength Training, refer to Chapter 3; My Wii Fit Plus, Chapter 4; Aerobics, Chapter 5; and Training Plus and Balance Games, Chapter 6.

What follows are some general navigation tips:

✔ Hover over an icon in a Training submenu to see the name of the exercise and how many times it's been attempted with your Mii. Unlike the original Wii Fit, all exercises are available to you from the outset, except for the three Strength Training Challenges, which are grayed out and will have to be unlocked.

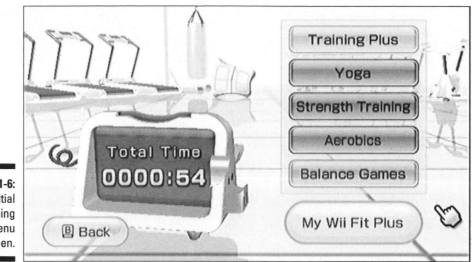

Figure 1-6:
The initial
Training
menu
screen.

✔ Click the + and − buttons at the top of the screen or press the same buttons on the Wii Remote in a Training submenu to go directly to the other training submenus.

✔ Click the Back button in the lower-left corner of a Training submenu or press the B button on your Wii Remote to go back to the Training menu.

✔ Click the Switch Trainer icon to toggle between the male and female trainer in the Yoga and Strength submenu.

✔ In the Yoga and Strength Training submenu, after you select an exercise, you can click Demo to watch a trainer explain how to do the chosen movement. Click the Skip button at any time to jump to a screen that allows you to get a more detailed view of the trainer performing the exercise. From this screen, you can rotate your viewpoint around the trainer by pressing A and moving the Wii Remote pointer around the screen. The 1 and 2 buttons on the Wii Remote allow you to zoom in and out, respectively. Click the Pause button on the screen to stop a trainer's movement and study its position, or click Restart to have the demonstration begin again. After you are ready to begin the activity, click the Start Workout button on the lower right of the screen. When you're performing an exercise, press up or down on the directional pad on your Wii Remote to change the camera angle focused on the trainer between front and rear to personalize your view.

✔ Switch between players by clicking the Switch! button on the bottom right of the screen in the Training Plus, Aerobics, and Balance Games submenus. You can select from any of the players on your system, including unregistered users, but these players won't build up Fit Credits, which we discuss shortly.

At any time during training, you can click the + button on your Wii Remote to bring up the Pause menu, which will give you the option to Continue, Retry, or Quit. Continue resumes the current activity, Retry restarts the current activity, and Quit brings you back to the Training menu. Keep in mind that if you Quit, you won't get any Fit Credits for the current activity. So, let's go over those Fit Credits.

Fit Credits and Fit Bank

Notice that cute little piggy bank with the display on the left of the Training menu? This is your Fit Bank or Fit Piggy, as it is often referred to in the game. When you engage in *Wii Fit Plus* activities, you are rewarded with Fit Credits, which get deposited into this Fit Bank. The number of Fit Credits earned varies based on how much time you spend performing an activity. Although the Fit Bank only keeps track of your daily earnings, you can see your cumulative counts by going to the Calendar screen, pressing the graph icon, and selecting Fit Credits; the Calendar screen is discussed in detail earlier in this chapter. As you accumulate Fit Credits, more advanced activities become unlocked, providing great motivation to stick with the program.

Besides storing your Fit Credits and looking cute, your Fit Bank serves another important purpose. After you complete an activity, the estimated number of calories used during that exercise will be presented to you and displayed on your Fit Bank, a feature that was lacking in the original Wii Fit.

If you are wondering how these calorie calculations are made, the *Wii Fit Plus* software uses a METs calculator. A MET, or metabolic equivalent of task, represents the intensity of an activity. For example, it takes 1 MET to sit still, which is considered your resting metabolic rate. Super Hula Hoop in *Wii Fit Plus* has a worth of 4 METs, which would be equivalent to a light walk or round of golf on foot. If you know the MET value of an activity, you can calculate the number of calories burned while performing that activity by using the following equation:

METs × Your Weight × Time (hours) × 0.48 = Calories Burned.

Keep in mind that all values for calories burned are estimates. The actual number of calories burned may be different due to factors such as your metabolic rate and efficiency of movement. Regardless, this caloric measure is a good way to get a sense of how much you may or may not be pushing yourself during your workout.

Wii Fit Plus Channel

You can check your profiles and *Wii Fit Plus* stats, and perform the Body Test without having to insert the game disc into your system by simply installing the *Wii Fit Plus* Channel. Do this at the Wii Fit Plaza, where you click on the Settings wrench icon at the upper right of the screen to bring up a submenu, then click on the Install Channel option. Click OK at the confirmation screen to install the *Wii Fit Plus* Channel on the Wii Menu. Click OK after the Save to the Wii System Memory prompt appears. After it's installed, click OK when you see Finished Saving. The next time you access the Wii Menu, you will see the new channel, as shown in Figure 1-7.

The *Wii Fit Plus* Channel takes up 109 blocks on your Wii's internal memory, so you need to ensure that you have sufficient space for a successful installation. Refer to the Wii Operations Manual that came with your console or *Wii For Dummies* by Kyle Orland (Wiley Publishing) for more on memory management.

Figure 1-7:
A typical *Wii Fit Plus* Channel view.

Warming Up and Cooling Down

Before you start doing any of the activities in *Wii Fit Plus,* the program reminds you to warm up; however, no warm-up activities are provided outside of Warm Up, found under the Lifestyle category of *Wii Fit Plus* Routines, which is described in Chapter 4. As a general rule, before beginning any type of physical activity, it is important to elevate your body temperature and get the muscle groups you'll be targeting moving. Contrary to popular belief, stretching is not recommended as part of your warm-up because stretching cold muscles can cause pulls and tears, potentially leading to serious injury. If you wish to stretch, do so at the end of your workout when your body has been put through its paces and is already warm, and be sure to stretch only within your limits.

The best way to warm up is with light aerobic exercise — just enough to break a sweat and test how your body is responding. This can include activities like jogging in place, jumping rope, or performing jumping jacks. If you'll be performing strength-based movements, it's a good idea to also warm up the general areas you'll be working, such as with push-ups for upper body or bodyweight squats for lower body. Whatever you do, keep the activities low impact and low stress. Generally speaking, a good warm-up should approximate the activity or activities you'll be performing and last only five to ten minutes, but feel free to adjust as needed to sufficiently elevate your body's temperature.

Chapter 2

Understanding Your Baseline

· ·

In This Chapter

▶ Finding your center of balance

▶ Controlling your body

▶ Determining your Wii Fit Age

▶ Setting goals

▶ Monitoring your progress

▶ Using a password

· ·

*W*hen following an exercise regime, determining your baseline physical fitness level and recording your progress may prove both challenging and time-consuming. This is likely the reason why many people don't bother to keep a fitness log. Yet, a record can be invaluable in identifying trends and assessing your overall progress. Fortunately, *Wii Fit Plus* makes the process simple. You can perform a series of tests, and *Wii Fit Plus* saves this information, which it then plots out for you in graphs for future reference. This format is certainly easier than reading chicken scratch on paper and it saves a few trees in the process. You can even record physical activities outside of the *Wii Fit Plus* program.

This chapter provides an overview of your center of balance and the Wii Fit Plus Balance and Mind and Body Tests that are used to assess it and your Wii Fit Age. We also explain your Body Mass Index (BMI) and weight assessments, review how to mark your results, and go about setting realistic goals. Guidance on navigating the many charts that track your progress is also provided.

Finding Your Center of Balance

Your *center of balance,* more commonly referred to as your *center of gravity,* is the point between the left and right sides of your body in which your body mass (weight) is considered to concentrate and through which gravity is enacting its constant downward force. It is this point that is working hard to keep you balanced. For most people, this point lies at roughly the level of the second sacral vertebra (S2), which is located in the lower part of the back just above the coccyx (tailbone) when standing upright, but it can vary based on your age, sex, build, posture, and whether you are supporting any external weight, such as a purse or shopping bag. It will also change depending on the position of your body and your movements. For example, your center of balance is lower when you bend your knees to perform the Rowing Squat under the Strength Training exercises and higher when you raise your arms to do the Half-Moon pose under the Yoga exercises (both of these are outlined in Chapter 3). The Balance Board has four Balance Sensors, which it uses to find and track your center of balance during most *Wii Fit Plus* activities; some activities just use the Wii Remote. Using the Remote allows you to make adjustments during the exercises, ensuring proper form and potentially helping you to improve your posture, which will prevent unnatural strain on your muscles, joints, and ligaments. To see if your posture and balance are improving, you can check your center of balance any time by taking the Body Test.

Body Test

The Body Test can be accessed by clicking Body Test on the lower left of the Calendar screen. This test has several components, including the Center of Balance Test, BMI, and the Mind and Body Control Tests. The Mind Tests are new to *Wii Fit Plus,* so unlike the original Wii Fit, your mental capabilities can also factor into your Wii Fit Age. If you are using *Wii Fit Plus* for the first time, you have to do all three to establish a baseline, as outlined in Chapter 1. On subsequent use, you can elect to do none; just the Center of Balance Test and BMI/weight assessment; or a complete assessment, including the Center of Balance Test, BMI/weight, and two of the Mind and Body Control Tests, both of which will be chosen for you at random.

If you want to establish your center of balance and BMI in under one minute, you can do so with the Simple Test, which appears in the Wii Fit Plaza after you select your Mii.

If you choose to do a complete assessment, your results will be used to determine your Wii Fit Age. The Body Test begins by prompting you to enter the weight of your clothes. You can choose Light (–2 lbs.), Heavy (–4 lbs.), or Other, which allows you to input a specific weight (up to ±7 lbs.) by pressing up and down on the directional pad on the Wii Remote. You can even input 0 if you are in the mood to exercise in the nude — hey, we aren't going to judge you! Inputting a weight for your clothes ensures you receive a more accurate measure of your bodyweight and BMI, provided you are good at estimating or like to weigh your clothes before you put them on in the morning. All silliness aside, if you are wearing a T-shirt and shorts, generally picking Light will suffice. If you are wearing sweats, selecting Heavy works better.

You can hone your ability to estimate weight by engaging in the Scale Challenge, which you can access after you click on the virtual Balance Board that hangs out in the Training Menu. Disguised as a mental challenge, this frantic and fun mini game has you placing objects on the Balance Board that equal the amount of weight given as closely and quickly as possible. After you are satisfied with your estimation, press A. *Wii Fit Plus* provides feedback on the level of your accuracy. You have 30 seconds to complete five rounds.

Center of Balance Test

When the game prompts you, stand on the Balance Board with your body straight and your feet spread equally apart with your toes slightly pointed out.

Relax your shoulders and hold still — think mime or statue. Following a three-second countdown, your balance on the left, right, front, and back of your body will be measured by the four Balance Board sensors.

If you fidget too much, the test will end prematurely and you will have to step off the Balance Board and start again. After the measuring is complete, which takes just a few seconds, your results are shown on the onscreen Balance Board by a red dot that traces a line showing the shifts that were detected in your center of balance. The *Wii Fit Plus* software will then mark a red dot where your average center of balance is located and provide you with a percentage measure for your right and left sides, as shown in Figure 2-1.

To mix things up, *Wii Fit Plus* occasionally asks you to close your eyes during the Center of Balance Test. If you can't help but sneak a peek, you will discover that the screen has turned black. If your balance is found to be way off — eyes open or shut — *Wii Fit Plus* administers a second test that is intended to make you more aware of your center of balance. Your current center of balance appears as a red dot on the onscreen Balance Board. The goal is to shift your weight accordingly so that you move the red dot into the blue circle in the center of the onscreen Balance Board and hold it there for three seconds.

If you find that the results of your Center of Balance Test fluctuate widely, this may have to do with your foot placement on the Balance Board. Make sure your left and right feet match; for example, one foot shouldn't be straight while the other is pointing out. You can use the contours on the Balance Board as a guide.

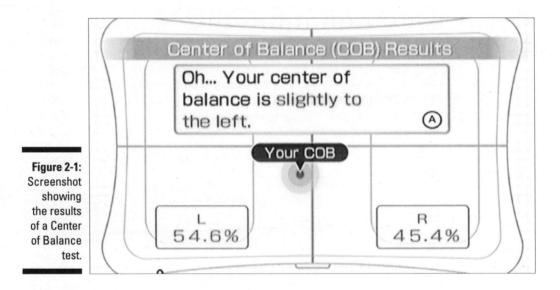

Figure 2-1: Screenshot showing the results of a Center of Balance test.

Body Mass Index (BMI)

During the Center of Balance Test, Wii Fit Plus also measures your weight and calculates your BMI, which it now shares with you. Figure 2-2 provides a glimpse of the BMI results screen. The Weight screen can be accessed by clicking on Weight at the bottom of the BMI screen.

Although *Wii Fit Plus* places a lot of emphasis on BMI, the *Wii Fit Plus* Instruction Booklet does point out three limitations.

✔ BMI is typically used as a measure of health in adults, so when BMI results are provided for a player between 3 and 19 years of age, it may not be as accurate, even though *Wii Fit Plus* was designed to allow BMI assessment in this age group. To ensure accuracy of this measure in children and teens, who may experience some serious growth spurts, it is important to keep their height information up-to-date. This can be done by clicking on the happy-face, word-balloon icon in the Calendar screen, selecting Edit Profile, and then clicking on the listed height and making the adjustment. Be sure to choose Save when you are done.

✔ BMI can't distinguish between muscle and fat, so if you are more muscular, your BMI may end up in the Overweight or even Obese range, and *Wii Fit Plus* will inflate your Mii to become heftier. Unfortunately, *Wii Fit Plus* has no means of accounting for muscle, so you'll just have to deal with a potentially untrue visual assessment. What's the big deal anyway, right? You know what you look like, and it isn't like Miis can be muscular or shapely anyway.

✔ BMI is not the only measure of health that counts. Your cholesterol levels (high-density lipoprotein, low-density lipoprotein, and triglycerides), blood pressure, blood sugar levels, heart rate, and numerous other factors are equally important, and these levels are affected by many factors, only one of which is weight or your BMI. So, even if you have a BMI of 22, which is considered to be the healthiest (people with this BMI are statistically less likely to get sick according to *Wii Fit Plus*), don't let that lull you into a false sense of security. Only a complete physical examination by a qualified physician can guarantee a completely clean bill of health.

So, why even bother with BMI? Despite its limitations, BMI is a reliable indicator of body fat for *most* people and is a simple tool that can be used to screen for weight categories that have a higher risk of health problems. Until there is a console that comes with a blood pressure cuff attachment and that can screen your blood — though we are not sure how much fun that would be — BMI will have to do. Certainly, you know your health better than anyone else and are the best judge of how meaningful your *Wii Fit Plus* BMI measure truly is.

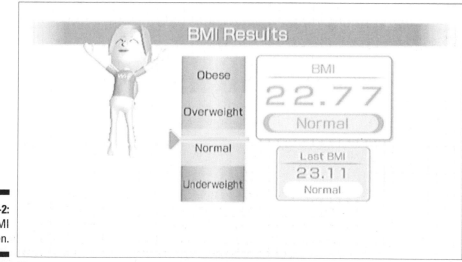

Figure 2-2:
The BMI
screen.

Controlling Your Body

To assess how adept you are at controlling your body, *Wii Fit Plus* has ten Mind and Body Control Tests that challenge your balancing abilities and assess your mental prowess. When you initially play *Wii Fit Plus,* you are just given the Basic Balance test, but on subsequent testing, two tests are chosen for you at random, some of which are more easily performed than others. Regardless, the information gleaned from these tests may help you ascertain whether you are favoring one side of your body over the other and how well your brain and body react to visual data and stimuli. The ten Mind and Body Control Tests, plus bonus, are as follows:

✔ **Agility Test:** Do you have the ability to shift your center of balance quickly and precisely? Find out with this test, which requires you to shift your weight in all directions on the Balance Board — front, back, left, and right — in a very controlled fashion to hit the blue boxes with the red dot that represents your center of balance, as demonstrated in Figure 2-3. You have 30 seconds to hit as many boxes as possible. This test becomes progressively more difficult; initially, there are several rounds with single boxes, followed by multiple boxes, and, ultimately, moving boxes.

Be sure to move your upper body forward and backward for this activity as well, as front and back shifts in balance (the sagittal plane of motion) are also required to get those boxes. Although it may be tempting to randomly move in any and every direction, use controlled movements to sharpen your proprioceptive sense, which is the unconscious awareness of the space that your body occupies. These exercises are especially good if you are accident prone like one of the authors of this book.

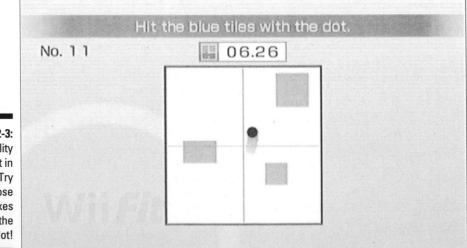

Figure 2-3: The Agility Test in action. Try to hit those blue boxes with the red dot!

✔ **Basic Balance Test:** Want to see how good you are at shifting your weight between the left and right sides of your body? If so, this test can provide some much-needed answers. The two onscreen vertical bars represent your left and right sides. As you shift your weight, the bars become filled in red, depending on how much pressure is being applied. Thus, if most of your weight is being put on your left side, the left vertical bar will be almost completely filled, whereas the bar on the right will be almost empty, as shown in Figure 2-4. You will also see blue rectangular areas on each of the vertical bars. The goal is to shift your weight so that each bar gets filled enough to reach the blue rectangular area, which turns yellow when you reach it, and then to hold that position for three seconds, at which point those elusive blue rectangles will change positions. You have five rounds to master.

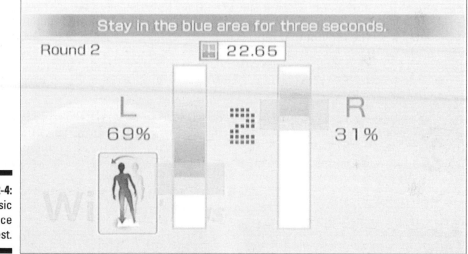

Figure 2-4:
The Basic
Balance
Test.

✔ **Dual Balance Test:** Are you adept at shifting your balance while also adjusting the position of your arms? You can find out with this activity, which is the Basic Balance Test with a twist. For this activity, you hold the Wii Remote with both hands out in front of you and follow the instructions for the Basic Balance Test, as previously outlined, while also adjusting the position of your Wii Remote so that it lines up with the blue bar that appears in the onscreen circle that represents your Wii Remote. This circle appears in the center of the screen between the vertical bars. After you successfully shift your balance and line up the Wii Remote, all blue bars turn yellow. You now have to hold steady for three seconds, after which you progress to the next round. You have 30 seconds to complete five rounds.

This test is one of the more challenging Mind and Body Tests. If you find you are having a tough time coordinating all movements, try to adjust your center of balance on the Balance Board first and then adjust your Wii Remote to match the position of the blue bar that appears in the onscreen circle that represents your Wii Remote.

✔ **Judgment Test:** Are you able to quickly process information and react appropriately? See how well your brain and body collaborate with this virtual twist on Simon Says, where you need to move your body to select numbers that are either less than or greater than a number designated by *Wii Fit Plus.* To start the test, you have to shift your center of balance so that the red dot appears in the blue circle on the center of the screen. A number in a green bubble appears onscreen. For example, if the number needs to be less than five, shift your center of balance to select it, as shown in Figure 2-5. If not, stay as still as a mouse. For the next number to appear, the red dot needs to move to the blue circle. See if you can get all 20 correct.

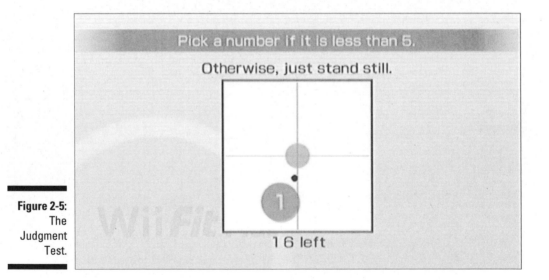

Figure 2-5:
The
Judgment
Test.

✔ **Memory Test:** Do you have the memory of an elephant? Find out with this test, which gives you 25 chances to compare the number in the center with the number to the right. If the number to the right is greater than the center number, you have to crush the center number by squatting to bring down the press that appears above it. If you don't want to crush that number, stay still or that press is going to come down. Initially, all of the numbers are visible, but eventually they will be covered up and you will have to recall what the numbers were.

✔ **Peripheral Vision Test:** How keen is your peripheral vision? Find out with this test, which is one of the more challenging Body Tests. The test starts by having you center your balance by adjusting your body so that the red dot appears in the middle blue circle. After you hold this position for three seconds, numbers will appear onscreen. You have to click on them in ascending order, from 1 to 10, while keeping the red dot in the blue circle. After you move the Wii Remote so that the cursor appears on top of the desired number, press A. Be sure not to move on the Balance Board. If the red dot migrates outside the blue circle, the numbers vanish and you will have to center yourself again on the board before the numbers will reappear.

If you have trouble with this test, you can hone your skills by doing Basic Run Plus, which requires you to use your peripheral vision. Basic Run Plus is found under Training Plus and is described in Chapter 6.

✔ **Prediction Test:** Are you able to predict obstacles that lie ahead of you? This 60-second test, which is reminiscent of Balance Bubble and Balance Bubble Plus (both are described in Chapter 6), requires you to shift your center of balance to the right or left to avoid hitting the walls and other obstacles, some of which are mobile. To complete the test, you have to look ahead and predict where the mobile obstacles are going to be when you reach them to avoid a collision. If an impact ensues, it's game over.

You can hone your prediction skills by training with Obstacle Course, Balance Bubble Plus, and Balance Bubble. The former two appear in Training Plus and the latter under Balance Games. Turn to Chapter 6 to find out more about these activities.

✔ **Single Leg Balance Test:** Can you stand on one leg for 30 seconds? Sounds simple doesn't it? After you select which leg you'd like to stand on, place it on the line in the middle of the Balance Board, lift your other leg off the Balance Board (you can rest it against the standing leg, if desired), and press A. The testing will now commence. You see an onscreen graph with two thin vertical borders, as shown in Figure 2-6. As you balance yourself, your frontal plane of motion (side-to-side balance) is illustrated by a red line that stems from a triangle (this represents your foot) resting on a horizontal red line (this represents the Balance Board) with a thin blue vertical line through the middle of it that extends from the top to the bottom of the graph (this represents the line through the middle of your Balance Board). The left and right sides are indicated on each side of the graph, and percentages for how much of your weight is distributed on both sides of your foot are provided. As the test progresses, those thin vertical borders become more prominent, allowing less wiggle room — if you go into the blue, it's game over.

If you are concerned about your stability, you can use an object or spotter for support. Just be sure to keep practicing so that you can eventually shed these aides.

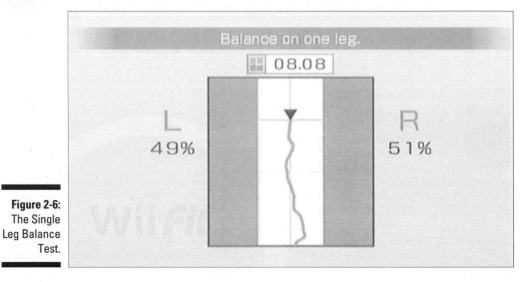

Figure 2-6:
The Single
Leg Balance
Test.

✔ **Stillness Test:** Can you remain as still as the Royal Guards who protect Buckingham Palace? Find out with this 30-second test (called the Steadiness Test in the original Wii Fit), which requires you to hold as still as possible — no fidgeting. That's it! Easy, right? Like an annoying tourist, *Wii Fit Plus* tries to distract you. A red dot designating your center of balance appears onscreen in a black and white grid, and after ten seconds, the grid starts to move. Don't follow it. Just keep your stance. In ten seconds, the dot and grid completely vanish. Keep holding still, because it isn't game over yet. After another ten seconds pass, testing is complete and your movements are revealed. Are you Guard material?

✔ **Walking Test:** Is there a spring in your step or is your gait off-kilter? This test reveals how well you are able to distribute your weight as you walk. *Wii Fit Plus* instructs you to stand with your feet spread equally apart and then walk in place for 20 steps; try to avoid any unnatural, exaggerated movements. Make sure to keep your feet in the textured squared-off sections of the Balance Board; otherwise you will look like a waddling duck and your steps may not register. The meter at the top of the screen counts your steps, and the onscreen foot that corresponds with the side being stepped on will turn red, enlarge, and have blue rings emanating from it as you take each step. That sounds ominous, doesn't it? Don't worry; your real feet won't take a beating with this activity. At the end, your balance for each side will be provided as a percentage. You also receive a percentage for your overall balance, and if you completed the activity before, the previously attained value will be provided as a point of reference.

The faster you go, the better your result will be; however, if you want a more accurate assessment of your balance while walking, a normal pace is the way to go.

✔ **Ultimate Balance Test:** This test is not a randomly generated test, but it fits in very well here. After you are all set up, you can access this test anytime from the Training Menu. Just click on the animated virtual Balance Board in the background; it may be throwing punches or jogging on one of the treadmills. After you click on it, you are asked: Would you like to take the Ultimate Balance Test? Once you click Yes, you will find that this activity is reminiscent of the Basic Balance Test, except that you now have to distribute your weight evenly. Although the blue bars are always aligned at the center (50 percent mark), they are now much thinner and will proceed to get even thinner as the test progresses through all three rounds. You have 60 seconds to get through the activity, and for each round, you have to stay within the blue area for three seconds. See if you can make it through. After you do, you can try to beat your time to get a new record. You have to hold your stance 50-50 for 60 demanding seconds to be considered a Master of Balance.

After you perform a Mind and Body Test, that test will become available for you to practice anytime by going to the My Wii Fit Plus Menu and clicking on the virtual Balance Board cavorting in the background.

Determining Your Wii Fit Age

After you complete the randomly selected Body Tests, *Wii Fit Plus* presents you with your Wii Fit Age, which drops down on the screen as a giant number after a suspenseful drum roll. Whether you and your Mii are left feeling elated or disappointed after all that flourish, you can't put too much stock in the number. Although the calculation takes your actual age into consideration, it is based predominantly on your performance on the Body Tests, and not even your BMI or weight are factored in.

Although the *Wii Fit Plus* instruction booklet suggests that your fitness goals can include lowering your Wii Fit Age, this is not an appropriate goal because your Wii Fit Age can fluctuate widely, even on the same day. Some Body Tests are easier than others, and until you master each of them, there may be vast differences in your Wii Fit Age, depending on which combination you get. So, although your Wii Fit Age is truly but a number, and is about as relevant an indicator of your health as a crystal ball is for telling your future, it sure can provide a laugh or two, and that is always good for your health.

Marking Your Results

After you complete a Body Test, be sure to record the result by stamping your calendar before you shut off the system or start training. Just point the Wii Remote at the highlighted date on the Calendar screen and press A. Initially, the only available stamp is that of an orange foot; however, as you continue taking Body Tests, seven more stamps will become available to you. What follows is how many Body Tests you need to take to unlock the stamps:

- OK: 2
- Star: 5
- Heart: 7
- Flower: 10
- Smiley Face: 14
- Clover: 22
- Mii: 30

To access these stamps, follow these steps:

1. **Click the smiling face icon at the upper right of the screen.**

2. **Select Change Design, and then hover over the stamp design you want.**

3. **Click A and then click OK.**

You can also unlock seven additional stamps for your pets. Initially, an orange paw print will be available.

If you want to use a new stamp design, be sure to change it before the Body Test. Even though you can retake the Mind and Body tests and update your results, you can't change the stamp on your calendar after it's been marked.

Setting Goals

Wii Fit Plus allows you to set weight-loss or weight-gain goals. After you set your goal, you are locked in for one week, unless you reach that goal earlier or want to create a new Mii or delete your user data. You can undertake the last option by clicking on the happy-face, word-balloon icon on the top right of the Calendar screen and then selecting Delete User Data. However, after you delete it, all of your data is gone forever.

Statistically, people with a BMI of 22 are said to be the least likely to get sick, and if your BMI is over 25, you may have increased health risks; however, as discussed earlier, BMI has considerable limitations. Don't obsess over a BMI goal — try to keep your weight-loss goals to one to two pounds per week. Your doctor can provide the best guidance, as he or she will be able to take your medical history into account.

Also, try to keep your goals realistic. We suggest setting smaller goals, as this will enhance motivation and effort. If you feel you're able to constantly improve, you're more likely to stick with your exercise program and be more enthusiastic about it. Bigger goals can feel overwhelming and unattainable, which may increase the chance that you'll throw in the towel before you've realized your full potential. Furthermore, accomplishing several smaller goals adds up to that big goal faster than you think.

If you start to build muscle, you may find your weight going up. This is because muscle weighs more than fat, and this should not be considered a bad thing. What matters most is how you feel. It truly is not all about the numbers, so don't be disheartened if you don't reach the goal you've set. It's the progress that counts, even if it's one more repetition on an exercise or being able to hold a yoga position for a few seconds longer.

Assessing and Comparing Your Results

To review changes in your BMI, weight, Wii Fit Age, Fit Credits, Waist, and Steps, click on the graph icon on the lower left of the Calendar screen, which pulls up a graph with tabs for each of these categories, as shown in Figure 2-7. Click on the desired tab to review your results. You can scroll through any of these graphs by pointing at the graph, pressing and holding the A button, and then moving your Wii Remote in the direction you want to scroll. You can also change the time point displayed for any of these graphs by clicking – or + in the Graph Display Area, which is located to the right directly below the calendar and to the left of your Mii.

The following list examines each of these tabs in greater detail.

✔ **BMI:** Initially, the horizontal axis lists the days of the current month and the vertical axis lists BMI. A triangular point shows your goal. The dates that Body Tests were taken are plotted out in a line graph, allowing you to see how close you are to reaching your goal and whether you've made any progress. If you hover over the points, the date and your BMI pop up in a black bubble. Clicking the + in the Graph Display Area allows you to assess the results between different points in time, including 1 week, 2 weeks, 1 month, 3 months, and 1 year. The results for 3 months and 1 year are provided as a scatter plot, which allows you to easily observe trends. Did your BMI go up in December? Maybe you got carried away eating too much delicious holiday fare and can make a mental note not to let that happen again.

✔ **Weight:** This chart is plotted the same way as BMI, except that the vertical axis now lists weights. Depending on what your goal is relative to your weight, you may not see the point indicating your goal on the graph, unless you click the + in the Graph Display Area and pick another vantage point, such as 2 weeks or 3 months. As with BMI, the scatter plot views provide a good overview of trends in your weight, allowing you to identify potential weight busters, such as the ice cream shop that opened for the season next to where you work that you started frequenting in April.

✔ **Wii Fit Age:** Because your Wii Fit Age may vary greatly (see Determining Your Wii Fit Age, earlier in this chapter), this measure may best be observed as a scatter plot by selecting the 3-month or 1-year view from the Graph Display Area. Although not a very relevant measure of your progress or fitness level, it may be interesting to compare your highs and lows.

✔ **Fit Credits:** When you pull up this graph, you see dates on the horizontal axis, units of time in minutes on the vertical axis, and a color-coded key for each category of activity available on *Wii Fit Plus.* Notice that these colors correspond to those on the Training Menu; however, an additional category at the very top of this key, called Activity Log, has a corresponding button to the right of the key. If you record any exercises or activities done outside of *Wii Fit Plus* to the Activity Log, these are also tracked here as a bar graph; you can track activities for babies and pets as well. If multiple activities are performed on a given day, the bar will be divided into color segments of varying size to indicate the activities performed and how long they were performed. From the Graph Display Area, you can pick 1 week, 2 weeks, and 1 month. The 1-month setting is the easiest to scroll through, but the bars become quite small and may be hard to read.

✔ **Waist:** This measure is not automatically recorded by *Wii Fit Plus,* and any waist measurement must be manually entered. You can do this by clicking Waist and then Record. All waist measurements are entered in inches. For tips on measuring your waist, turn to Chapter 1. *Wii Fit Plus* allows you to track waist measurements for babies and pets as well.

✔ **Steps:** As with waist measurements, Steps are manually recorded. The ability to log your steps in *Wii Fit Plus* is useful if you use a pedometer. If you are considering purchasing one, turn to Chapter 13 for guidance on what to look for. If you already own a pedometer, strive for 10,000 steps a day — a common fitness goal. Wii Fit Plus allows you to keep track of steps for babies and pets as well. We aren't sure why you'd want to track baby steps, but if your dog or cat is in serious need of a diet, this feature may be useful. You can purchase pet pedometers at select retailers.

Activity Log

To add an activity to the Activity Log, press the Activity Log button. Press A when you see "You can record exercises and activities done outside *Wii Fit Plus* in your Activity Log," and then click on Yes when you see "Do you want to record an activity in your Activity Log?" You will then have to select an activity type, Light, Normal, or Hard. If you are unsure how your activity ranks, you can click on Examples for each of these to get an idea. After you make your selection, just click on the up and down arrows for hours and minutes as desired and press OK. You will then receive a summary of what was added, followed by the question "Would you like to add another activity?" Pick Yes or No, depending on what you'd like to do.

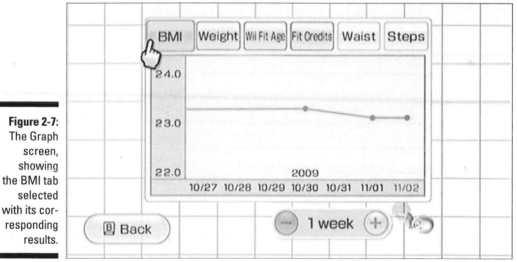

Figure 2-7:
The Graph screen, showing the BMI tab selected with its corresponding results.

Although the Fit Credits graph shows how much time you are investing in each type of *Wii Fit Plus* activity, it won't help you ascertain whether your performance on individual exercises is improving. Although the star ranking you receive after completing an exercise serves as a good indicator, as you will also see previous records and results, the best indicator is the ease with which you are able to perform an exercise. So, if at first your legs turned to jelly after squeezing out five Rowing Squats, but after some work you are able to do ten with relative ease, you've made a lot of progress!

Want to see how you performed on a past Body Test? Get a replay by clicking on the desired stamped date on the Calendar screen.

Locking and Unlocking Your Results

The Wii Fit Plaza has a graph that displays your BMI and that of all the Miis you have registered on your system, offering a point of comparison with other players. You can also access everyone's Fit Credits — that is, unless you want to hide your results and keep anyone else from accessing or playing as your Mii. Here is how:

1. **Click the happy-face, word-balloon icon at the top right of the Calendar screen, select Edit Profile, and click the None button next to Password.**

   Wii Fit Plus now asks you to set a password. Just click Yes.

2. **After you set your 4-digit password, click OK.**

3. **Reenter the password for verification and click OK.**

   You are notified that your password has been set.

4. **After you click A, you return to your profile and see four asterisks next to Password.**

5. **Click Save and your profile is now secure.**

   You can just click Back until you get to the Calendar screen.

Should you have a change of heart and want to undo the password, click the happy-face, word-balloon icon at the Calendar screen, choose Edit Profile, and click on the asterisks next to Password. A Change Password? prompt appears. Click Remove and then Yes when you see "Remove password." After you click Save, you are password-free.

Although you should select a password you will remember, such as a PIN or the last four digits of your Social Security number, there is no need to fret if you forget. Just keep entering the possibilities, and after four or five attempts, *Wii Fit Plus* will ask if you are really the person whose Mii you are trying to access. Assuming you are, click A. You will now be given a security question, such as "What is your height?" If you answer correctly, your Mii will become accessible, and you can go into the User Settings and change your password or remove it altogether. Of course, if the people you are trying to hide your information from also know very basic facts about you, such as height and date of birth, they can just as easily unlock your Mii, regardless of what your password is. Although a password may keep some prying eyes away, you are not guaranteed that your information will remain private.

Chapter 3

Getting Fit with Yoga and Strength Training

· ·

In This Chapter

▶ Getting started with yoga and strength training

▶ Understanding yoga

▶ Mastering the yoga poses

▶ Working your body with strength training

· ·

*I*t may seem unusual for us to cover yoga and strength training in the same chapter, but we have two reasons for doing so. The exercises we highlight in this chapter are what make *Wii Fit Plus* the excellent fitness software that it is, and yoga and strength training actually have a lot in common, with both activities helping you develop strength and increase endurance. Yoga does this by stretching the muscles by holding poses, while strength training builds the muscles through strenuous, repetitive motions, also known as *reps*.

The first part of this chapter focuses on yoga. In this section, we review the benefits of deep breathing and how to do it the right way. We also provide step lists for all the poses and include the Sanskrit/Hindi terms whenever possible in case you ever want to take a yoga class. In the strength training section, we discuss how bodyweight moves can effectively target all your major muscle groups and provide you with step lists for each of the strength-training exercises. Images of select yoga poses and strength-training exercises are also provided throughout. Of course, you can watch demos of any of the yoga and strength-training exercises being performed while you are working out with *Wii Fit Plus* by selecting Demo after you choose your activity. For more details on navigating menus, turn to Chapter 1. Let's get started!

Getting Started

The yoga and strength-training activities are accessed from the Training menu. Follow these steps to get started:

1. **To start yoga or strength-training activities, click the blue Yoga button or green Strength Training button on the Training menu.**

2. **When you are at your desired exercise selector menu, pick the activity you want to perform.**

   After you select an activity, you see the exercises summary information, including the metabolic equivalent of task (MET) value and equipment needed, and have three options: Back, Demo, and Start.

   • Selecting Back returns you to the Yoga or Strength Training exercise selector menu.

   • Selecting Demo activates a quick demonstration on performing the activity.

   • Selecting Start proceeds directly into training at the Activity Level indicated (Yoga does not have different activity levels, but Strength Training does with the number of reps), unless this is your first time selecting the activity, at which point you'll automatically watch a quick demonstration.

3. **For Strength Training, after you unlock more reps for an activity, you can select that activity level by pressing the + and − buttons on your Wii Remote or by clicking on the onscreen + and − buttons.**

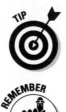

Any time during an exercise, you can press + on the Wii Remote to access the Pause menu, which gives you the option to Continue playing the current session, Retry (this restarts the activity), or Quit, which stops the activity and returns you to the Yoga or Strength Training Exercise selector menu.

Before starting any exercise program, consulting with a physician is wise. This is especially important if you have any of the conditions listed in the contraindications section of Table 3-1. After you have your physician's approval and are ready to begin, make sure that you take the time to warm up. Although the yoga poses in particular may appear gentle enough not to necessitate this, they can be demanding on your joints, ligaments, and muscles. By warming up, you are slowly raising your body temperature (hence the term "warming up"), which increases the flexibility of these structures and prevents tears, strains, and sprains. For more on warming up, turn to Chapter 1.

Understanding Yoga

You can try numerous yoga styles, but a fundamental goal of each is to unify the mind, body, and spirit through a series of poses (referred to by yogis as *asanas*), meditation, and breathing. Although *Wii Fit Plus* doesn't get into the meditative or spiritual aspects of this discipline, it provides a good introduction to some of the more common poses that can help you improve your balance, posture, and flexibility. *Wii Fit Plus* also helps you learn how to breathe properly, allowing you to maximize the fat-burning potential of each movement.

Deep Breathing, referred to by yogis as *pranayama,* is the first choice on the Yoga exercise selector menu, and for good reason. Breathing is something you do 15 times per minute on average, or approximately 22,000 times daily, and is one of those activities you rarely think about, but can have great health benefits if done properly. Deep breathing has been found to reduce stress, lower blood pressure, ward off or control panic attacks, boost immunity, and increase metabolic rate, so learning how to master this skill is worthwhile.

Follow these steps:

1. **Stand with your feet shoulder-width apart on the Balance Board and place your hands on your abdomen, roughly by your navel.**

   A blue circle, which will shrink and expand, encompasses your virtual trainer.

2. **Slowly inhale through your nose as the blue circle shrinks and exhale through your nose as it expands.**

   Alternately, you can also try inhaling through your nose and exhaling through your mouth.

3. **Relax your stomach after exhalation to let the air back in naturally upon inhalation.**

   Try to keep the red dot in the yellow center of the balance zone on the screen.

4. **Repeat for the full number of repetitions.**

Although it may seem like there is no correct way to breathe, many of us are shallow breathers and, therefore, are not oxygenating our cells as optimally as we could be, which can reduce performance. To determine if you are a shallow breather, place your hand on your abdomen after exhaling and then take a normal breath. If you don't feel your abdomen expand, you are likely only using your *intercostals* — the muscles between the ribs — rather than your diaphragm to draw in air. If you discover that this is the case, try performing the deep-breathing exercise a few times daily with or without your *Wii Fit Plus*.

Mastering the Yoga Poses

Wii Fit Plus offers a total of 18 poses, which are listed in Table 3-1. When doing the poses, always pay attention to your center of balance and your breathing to optimize performance and prevent injuries. Your center of balance is tracked by the red dot that appears in the yellow balance zone on the screen. If the red dot exits the yellow zone, it indicates that your balance is off, and the virtual trainer will offer guidance and encouragement to help you correct for it. Your breathing is monitored by the blue circle that surrounds your virtual trainer. As the blue circle shrinks, slowly inhale through your nose, and as the circle expands, slowly exhale through your nose.

If you want to add a spiritual aspect to your yoga routine, try taking the name of the poses literally. Envision yourself as the warrior, cobra, tree, or whatever pose you happen to be doing.

Table 3-1 **Master List of Yoga Exercises**

Exercise*	Sanskrit/Hindi Name	Target	Purpose	Pose Type	Menu Row	Potential Contraindications**	Advanced User?***
Deep Breathing	Pranayama	Entire Body	Improves Metabolism	Two-legged	First	None, but discontinue if you become light-headed, tired, or irritable	No
Half-Moon	Ardha Chandrasana	Waist	Increase Flexibility	Two-legged	First	Low blood pressure, headache, diarrhea, insomnia, varicose veins	No
Warrior	Virabhadrasana	Thighs and Hips	Aligns Pelvis	Two-legged	First	High blood pressure, diarrhea	No
Tree	Vrksasana	Legs and Back	Strengthens	One-legged	First	Headache, insomnia, high or low blood pressure	No
Sun Salutation	Surya Namaskar	Arms and Thighs	Increases Flexibility	Two-legged	First	High blood pressure, pregnancy, chronic back problems	No
Standing Knee	N/A****	Thighs	Increases Flexibility	One-legged	Second	Pregnancy, knee and chronic back problems	No
Palm Tree	Talasana	Calves, Ankles, and Back	Strengthens and Improves Balance	Two-legged	Second	High or low blood pressure	No
Chair	Utkatasana	Back, Legs, and Abs	Strengthens and Improves Balance	Two-legged	Second	Headache, insomnia, low blood pressure	No
Triangle	Trikonasana	Lower Body and Waist	Strengthens	Two-legged	Second	High or low blood pressure, diarrhea, headache, heart or neck conditions	No
Downward-Facing Dog	Adho Mukha Svanasana	Back	Stretches and Strengthens	Floor	Second	High blood pressure, pregnancy, diarrhea, carpal tunnel syndrome	No

(continued)

Table 3-1 (continued)

Exercise*	Sanskrit/Hindi Name	Target	Purpose	Pose Type	Menu Row	Potential Contraindications**	Advanced User?***
Dance	Natarajasana	Hips and Spine	Improves Balance and Aligns	One-legged	Third	Low blood pressure	Yes
Cobra	Bhujangasana	Back	Improves Posture	Floor	Third	Carpal tunnel, headache, back injury, pregnancy	Yes
Bridge	Setu Bandha Sarvangasana	Torso and Hips	Strengthens	Floor	Third	Neck injury	Yes
Spinal Twist	Supta Matsyendrasana	Back and Pelvis	Stretches and Aligns	Floor	Third	Back or spine injury	Yes
Shoulder Stand	Sarvangasana	Abs and Back	Strengthens	Floor	Third	High blood pressure, menstruation, pregnancy, and ear, eye, and neck disorders	Yes
Spine Extension***	Balasana	Shoulders, Legs, and Waist	Strengthens	Two-legged	Fourth	Back or neck injury, pregnancy, high blood pressure	Yes
Gate	Parighasana	Side Torso, Hamstrings, Calves, Shoulders, and Abdomen	Stretches and relieves tension	Floor	Fourth	Knee injury	Yes
Grounded V	Navasana	Abs	Strengthens	Floor	Fourth	Asthma, diarrhea, headache, heart problems, low blood pressure, menstruation, pregnancy, neck injury	Yes

*Yoga poses have many variations, depending on the yoga style; therefore, if you were to take a yoga class, you may find these poses performed slightly differently from the Wii Fit Plus versions. For instance, there is a Warrior (Virabhadrasana) I, II, and III, of which the Wii Fit Plus offers Warrior II.

**This list includes the most common contraindications for each pose, but these are by no means the only ones. Before starting any exercise, it is important to consult with your physician, especially if you have any of the conditions on the list.

***Advanced User activities are those deemed to be more challenging by Wii Fit Plus.

****N/A indicates non-applicable and denotes an activity for which we could find no Sanskrit/Hindi name equivalent.

Standing poses

Wii Fit Plus's ten standing poses can be broken down into roughly three types: stretch, two-legged balance, and one-legged balance. Of course, stretch poses require balance and balance poses require stretching, but this categorization emphasizes the primary challenge and objective of the exercises.

Stretch poses

Stretching is important for everyone, but is especially critical for us pencil pushers who spend a great deal of time seated in front of a computer on a daily basis. Sitting for extended periods of time puts considerable stress on our spines, resulting in poor posture and muscle tension, stiffness, or pain in the shoulders, neck, and back. By stretching on a daily basis, you will alleviate the stress on your spine, helping to prevent structural degradation. Stretching also promotes blood flow throughout the body, which can alleviate mental stress and anxiety and is important for muscular health and development. The *Wii Fit Plus* yoga stretch moves effectively target the spine and are designed to increase flexibility. Some of the gentler poses are also good as warm-ups.

Half-Moon

The Half-Moon *(Ardha Chandrasana)* is a side stretch pose that targets your waist muscles and can improve your posture and digestive health. After you learn this pose on *Wii Fit Plus,* you can easily perform it anywhere, even a transoceanic flight. Follow these steps:

1. **Stand with your feet together on the Balance Board and raise your arms above you head, interlocking your fingers.**

2. **Bend your upper body to the left and hold the pose.**

   Make sure to follow the breathing cues and keep the red dot in the yellow balance zone.

If you master this pose or want to try a variation, keep one arm down at your side while extending the other arm above your head. Then bend your upper body in the direction of the nonextended arm and hold the pose. Be sure to follow the same breathing cues.

Sun Salutation

The Sun Salutation *(Surya Namaskar)* stretches your arms, thighs, and spine. Generally, this pose consists of a series of 12 postures that are performed as a sequence, with each posture flowing into the next. *Wii Fit Plus*'s Sun Salutation consists of the first three of these postures. Perform the pose by following these steps:

1. **Stand with your feet together on the Balance Board and raise your arms overhead in a steady motion, reaching as far back as possible.**

   You feel as though you are saluting the sun.

2. **While slowly exhaling, bend forward and touch your toes with both hands. If necessary, bend your knees slightly.**

3. **Hold the pose for the duration, following the breathing cues and maintaining the red dot in the yellow balance zone.**

Triangle

The Triangle *(Trikonasana)* strengthens your lower body and works your waist. Follow these steps:

1. **Stand with your feet together on the Balance Board and move your right leg off the Balance Board behind you so that your feet are roughly 3½ to 4 feet apart.**

   Your right foot should be pointing to the right at 90 degrees, and your left and right heels should be aligned.

2. **Raise your right arm above your head while keeping your left arm at your side.**

3. **Reach for your left leg with your right hand and raise your left arm straight into the air so that it is in line with the tops of your shoulders.**

   The fingers on your left hand should be separated and your head should be in a neutral position or turned so that you are looking at your left thumb.

4. **Push firmly with your heels and toes so that you are putting 60 percent of your weight on your front leg.**

   You know that you have achieved this when the red bar is maintained in the blue zone.

5. **Hold the pose for the duration, making sure to follow the breathing cues and then repeat with the other leg.**

In the mood for a variation? Instead of raising your arm straight into the air, stretch it over the back of the top ear. Your arm will be parallel to the floor and both arms will form a backward "C."

Spine Extension

The Spine Extension *(Balasana)* works your shoulders, legs, upper arms, and waist. It is considered an advanced pose, but it isn't as difficult as some of the poses that are considered non-advanced, especially if you follow the tip for this exercise. Follow these steps:

1. **Place your right foot on the Balance Board and your left foot behind you so that your heels are in line with each other and you have a wide base.**

2. **As you inhale, raise your hands up along your sides and bring your palms together above your head.**

3. **Release and bring your hands together behind your back with your palms together and fingers pointing up.**

   Relax your neck and shoulders as you expand your chest.

4. **Exhale and slowly bend your upper body forward, making sure to bend from the hips and not your back, as shown in Figure 3-1.**

   Hold the pose so that you are comfortable and your ability to breathe is not impaired.

5. **With your hips parallel to the floor, pull your chin into your chest and stretch your neck. Breathe slowly, and as you exhale, see if you can bend deeper.**

6. **Inhale as you raise your upper body and exhale as you bring your hands back to your sides.**

7. **Switch legs on the Balance Board and repeat.**

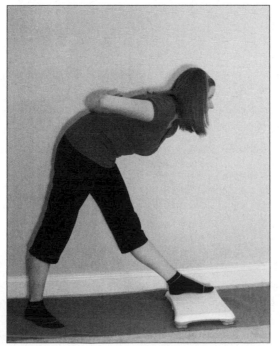

Figure 3-1:
Spine
Extension
apex.

If it is too difficult to bring your hands together behind your back, cross your arms behind your back instead.

Two-legged balance

Two-legged balance poses allow you to keep both feet on the ground, but they still put your balancing abilities to the test, whether by having you balance yourself on your toes or by having you shift your weight on the Balance Board. These poses help prepare you for the more complicated one-legged balance moves and are generally easier to master.

Warrior

There are three variations of the Warrior pose, called *Virabhadrasana* I, II, and III by yogis. *Wii Fit Plus* offers Virabhadrasana II. This pose, which is reminiscent of a fencing lunge, strengthens your thighs and hips and helps align your pelvis, improving your posture. Follow these steps:

1. **Stand with your feet together on the Balance Board and move your right leg off the Balance Board behind you, so that your feet are roughly 3½ to 4 feet apart.**

   Your right foot should be pointing to the right at 90 degrees, and your left and right heel should be aligned.

2. **Raise your arms so that they are parallel to the floor and reach them out to the sides.**

   Your shoulder blades should be open, your palms down, and your face looking forward.

3. **Bend your left knee over your left ankle, so that your shin is perpendicular to the floor.**

   Anchor this movement by maintaining weight on your front leg so that the red bar remains in the blue area for the designated time.

4. **Repeat with your right leg.**

If you are struggling to maintain your balance, try decreasing the distance between your feet. On the other hand, if you've mastered this pose, you can challenge yourself further by increasing the distance between your feet. In either case, make sure that the knee of the leg on the Balance Board is still over your heel and not your toes.

Palm Tree

The Palm Tree pose on *Wii Fit Plus* is a variation of the standard *Talasana*. This pose will strengthen your ankles and stretch your back. By stretching your spine vertically, it may straighten any minor curves, improving posture.

The pose is especially good at relieving tension, so if you are feeling stressed, follow these steps:

1. **Stand on the Balance Board with your feet approximately shoulder-width apart and feet turned slightly out.**

2. **Slowly raise your arms above your head so that your palms are facing out.**

3. **Raise your heels off the Balance Board and move your arms behind you so that your palms continue to face out.**

   You may vaguely feel like Kate Winslet catching the breeze in Titanic.

4. **Hold the pose for the duration, making sure to follow the breathing cues and keep the red dot in the yellow balance zone.**

Chair

The Chair pose *(Utkatasana)* is reminiscent of the rowing squat, which is described later in this chapter, and works the same muscles — back, legs, and abs. Master the Chair by following these steps:

1. **Start with your feet shoulder-width apart on the Balance Board.**

2. **Raise your arms in front of you so that your palms are down while simultaneously lifting your heels off the Balance Board so that you are standing on your toes.**

3. **Lower yourself so that your knees are bent.**

   You feel like you are sitting in an imaginary chair.

4. **Hold the pose for the duration while following the breathing cues and maintaining the red dot in the yellow balance zone.**

If you are struggling to maintain your balance, try a more traditional *Utkatasana* by keeping your feet flat on the Balance Board, instead of performing the pose while on your toes.

One-legged balance

Unless you are a flamingo, standing on one leg doesn't come naturally. However, as the old adage goes, practice makes perfect, so it pays to be persistent. One-legged poses are especially good at helping you become more in tune with your body because they require a great deal of concentration. Even if these poses seem intimidating, don't be afraid to give them a try. If you are concerned about losing your balance, try performing the moves with the Balance Board placed next to a wall or see if someone can spot you.

A distracted or restless mind can contribute to poor balance. Maintain your focus by locking your gaze on a point in front of you, and make sure you breathe deeply through your diaphragm (see the section on deep breathing in this chapter). If you still have trouble maintaining your balance, see if you can find someone to spot you.

Tree

The Tree (Vrksasana) is the quintessential yoga pose. This pose tests your ability to maintain your balance and strengthens your thighs, calves, ankles, and back. Try this pose by following these steps:

1. **Start with your feet shoulder-width apart on the Balance Board.**

2. **Pick up your right leg and grab your right ankle with your right hand.**

3. **Place your right foot as far up your left leg as possible, making sure your toes are pointing down.**

   Don't worry if you can't lift your leg very high; just place your foot at a comfortable level and try to focus on maintaining your balance for the duration of the pose. Your center of balance will be tracked by the red dot on the screen, which you should strive to keep in the yellow balance zone.

4. **Press your hands together in front of you at chest level, so that they assume the prayer position and raise your arms above your head.**

5. **Hold the pose until prompted to finish.**

6. **Repeat with your left leg.**

Perform this move wearing pants, rather than shorts, which provides traction and prevents your foot from sliding down your bare leg. Another way to help keep your foot locked into place is to actively press your leg into the sole of your foot while at the same time pressing your foot into your leg. After you can hold this pose for more than a few seconds, you can further challenge yourself by trying it with your eyes closed.

Standing Knee

This pose increases flexibility in your thighs. Perform the pose by following these steps:

1. **Start with your legs close together on the Balance Board.**

2. **Slowly lift your right leg to chest height, or as high as you can comfortably get it.**

3. **Hold your right knee with both hands and focus on maintaining your balance.**

4. **Repeat with your left leg.**

Dance

This move, also called *Natarajasana,* is quite elegant and reminiscent of a ballet move. Although *Wii Fit Plus* indicates this move can tone your hips and align your spine, it is actually a full body stretch that targets your shoulders, chest, abdomen, and legs. This pose is considered an advanced pose, and it may be a good idea to have a spotter around the first time you attempt it. Follow these steps:

1. **Stand with your feet together on the Balance Board.**

2. **Raise your right leg behind you and grab your foot with your right hand, bringing your right foot up to your buttocks (your knee will be bent), and raise your left hand above your head so that your palm faces outward.**

3. **Slowly lift your right foot up and back, extending away from your torso so that your right thigh is parallel to the floor, while at the same time stretching your left arm forward in front of you, as shown in Figure 3-2.**

    Your arm should be parallel to the floor with your palm facing down and your fingers pointed forward.

4. **Repeat with your left leg.**

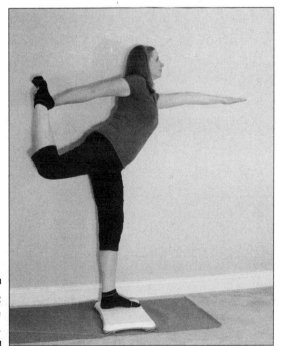

Figure 3-2:
Dance pose
apex.

If you can't grab your foot, you can try using a belt or other strap to hold it. Remember, you can always slow down and take the pose at your own pace.

Floor poses

Wii Fit Plus offers seven poses that are performed on the floor, only three of which use the Balance Board. These poses stretch and increase strength, but because most of them are not monitored, it is especially important to proceed with the moves cautiously and stretch only within your limits. These poses are best performed on an exercise mat. If you don't already own one, turn to Chapter 13 for some recommendations.

Downward-Facing Dog

The Downward-Facing Dog *(Adho Mukha Svanasana)* is a common yoga pose that targets your back while stretching your whole body. This pose is thought to relieve sinusitis, headaches, and constipation. However, if you suffer from high blood pressure or are suffering from a headache, it is advised that you support your head on a bolster or block so that your ears are level between your arms. This pose uses the Balance Board. Follow these steps:

1. **Get on all fours with your hands on the Balance Board, about shoulder-width apart, and your knees directly under your hips.**

2. **Exhale while you lift your hips as high as possible and straighten your arms and legs.**

   Try to distribute your weight evenly between your hands and feet; if you are successful doing this, the red bar on the screen remains in the blue area.

3. **Hold the pose for the duration, making sure to follow all breathing cues.**

If you want to challenge yourself further, try raising one of your legs so that it is parallel to the line of your torso. Hold this pose as long as possible and then perform it again, raising the opposite leg.

Cobra

Don't be fooled by the Cobra's *(Bhujangasana)* seeming simplicity. This pose is considered an advanced user pose. The Cobra is highly effective in stretching and strengthening the back muscles, helping to improve your posture. No Balance Board is required for this activity. Follow these steps to do the Cobra:

1. **Lie face down with your forearms on the floor and your chest open.**

   Your legs should be spread behind you.

2. **While inhaling, extend your elbows and lift your upper body off the floor.**

Don't be discouraged if you can't raise your upper body that far, and above all, don't force the backbend. Finding a height that is comfortable for you will prevent back strain. To do this, take your hands off the floor for a moment. The height you achieve by doing so is through extension, preventing an exaggerated bend that can result in injury. Another option is to remain in the Sphinx pose, which is the first step in the Cobra pose and is considered the "infant of backbends." If you remain in Sphinx pose, make the most of it by lightly lifting your belly away from the floor to create a dome that rounds up toward your lower back. This move is subtle, and you should not suck your belly in to achieve it.

Bridge

The Bridge pose *(Setu Bandha Sarvangasana)* is a more advanced backbend than the Cobra, and is considered an advanced user pose. The Bridge strengthens the torso and hips while stretching the neck and chest. If you are concerned about injuring your neck, consider placing a thickly folded blanket or towel under your shoulders for protection. This pose is performed sans Balance Board. Follow these steps:

1. **Lie face up with your knees bent, arms at your sides, and your feet flat on the floor as close to your buttocks as possible.**

2. **As you exhale, lift your hips off the floor until your thighs are roughly parallel to the floor.**

3. **Keep your knees directly over your heels and make sure your thighs and inner feet are parallel.**

   Your thighs should not touch.

   Your virtual trainer instructs you to hold the pose for 30 or 40 seconds, but you should only hold it for as long as is comfortable.

If you are looking to be more active, you can try lifting your hips up while slowly exhaling and rolling your body back down one vertebra at a time while slowly inhaling. If, on the other hand, you want to try a variation to the static Bridge, clasp your hands below your pelvis after you lift your hips off the floor.

Spinal Twist

The Spinal Twist, often referred to as *Jathara Parivrtti,* has many variations. The version *Wii Fit Plus* offers stretches your back and helps align your pelvis. Although the pose sounds menacing and uncomfortable, it is meant to be relaxing. However, the Spinal Twist is an advanced user pose. Concentrate on your breathing throughout the pose to optimize its restorative effects. Put your Balance Board aside and follow these steps:

1. **Lie face up on the floor, with your right arm stretched out to your side at shoulder height.**

2. **While exhaling, bend your right knee and use your left hand to guide and hold it down on your left side.**

   Be sure to release any tension from your hips and let your leg rest where it feels comfortable.

3. **Turn your head to the right and try to keep your right shoulder on the floor.**

   You can feel the stretch from your hips through your back.

Shoulder Stand

This pose, which is perhaps the most advanced of all *Wii Fit Plus* yoga poses, offers an inversion and strengthens the abs and back while aligning the legs. Because the Shoulder Stand *(Sarvangasana)* has the highest risk for injury, respecting your limits is necessary. One precaution you can take is to place a folded blanket or towel on the mat for your upper back and shoulders to rest on (your head and neck will be on the mat, not the blanket or towel), which helps prevent your neck from being injured when you raise your legs and bear your weight into the floor. The Balance Board is not used for this pose. Follow these steps:

1. **Lie face up on the floor with your arms at your sides, ensuring that your head and spine are aligned.**

2. **Lift both legs upon inhaling and then lift your back.**

3. **Bend your elbows and use your hands to support your back.**

   The higher up you place your hands, the straighter your pose will be.

4. **Straighten your body as you raise your legs toward the ceiling, using your shoulders for support, as demonstrated in Figure 3-3.**

   Keep your breathing slow and deep for the duration of the pose.

5. **To come out of this posture, gradually lower your hands to the floor, pressing your arms and palms into the mat for support.**

6. **Contract your abdomen while slowly lowering your upper back and finally buttocks back onto the mat.**

7. **To finish, lower your legs while pressing your lower spine into the mat.**

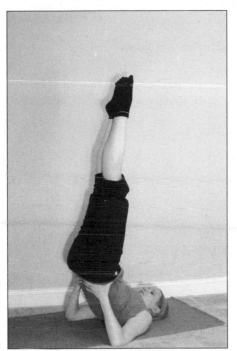

Figure 3-3:
Shoulder
Stand apex.

Gate

This Gate pose *(Parighasana),* considered an advanced user pose, opens the shoulders and stretches your hamstrings, spine, sides of the torso, and the muscles connecting the ribs, which are known as the intercostals. Because it elongates the intercostals, this pose allows the rib cage to move more freely, increasing the capacity of the lungs to draw in breath. As a result, the Gate pose is thought to be especially good for those with respiratory problems, such as asthma. Grab your Balance Board and follow these steps:

1. **Face left, go down on one knee, and put your right foot on the Balance Board.**

2. **Raise your left arm straight and extend your right hand over your knee, making sure to keep your left arm and thigh perpendicular to the floor.**

3. **Exhale and slowly lower your upper body to the right. Place your right hand on your ankle and expand the left side of your rib cage, as shown in Figure 3-4.**

   Try to distribute 30 percent of your weight to the right and hold this pose for 30 seconds while you breathe.

4. **Inhale and come back to the starting position. Exhale and drop your hand.**

5. **Stand up and repeat with your left leg.**

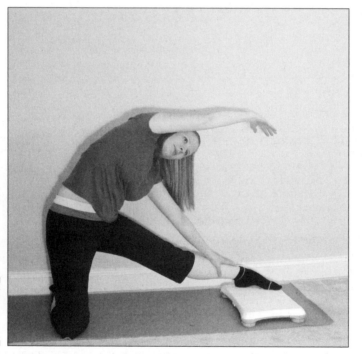

Figure 3-4:
Gate pose
apex.

Grounded V

This Grounded V pose is similar to the yoga Boat pose *(Navasana),* which is outlined in Chapter 11, except that you keep your hands behind you for stability instead of stretched out toward your legs. As the name of the pose implies, you will be making a V-shape with your body. This pose can be challenging and is considered an advanced user pose. For this pose, you are seated on the Balance Board. This activity is great at targeting your core. Follow these steps:

1. **Sit on the Balance Board and place your hands behind you for support.**

2. **Bring your legs together and exhale as you lift them up.**

   If you need to, bend your knees, but keep your calves parallel to the floor. Keep your back straight and concentrate on your abdomen. Hold this pose for 30 to 40 seconds as you breathe.

3. **Exhale and slowly bring your legs down to the starting position.**

Beginning Strength Training

When you think of strength training, you may envision a sweaty, grunting behemoth with bulging biceps throwing weights around at a gym. Yet there are numerous ways to effectively strength train without using weights. The method that *Wii Fit Plus* uses is body-weight training. Many people assume that body-weight training is not effective because the moves appear to be too simple to be of much value. To see firsthand why this is not the case, we suggest you get on the floor and try to do a push-up. How easy was it? If you haven't done a push-up since high school gym class, you may find it was quite challenging. Body-weight training helps you get strong relative to your own body weight and forces you to be very self-aware. You are not concentrating on moving a weight through space, but have to be cognizant of how you are moving your own body through space.

Wii Fit Plus offers 15 strength-training exercises and three challenges, as shown in Table 3-2. By showing you where your center of balance actually is versus where it should be, *Wii Fit Plus* ensures that you hit all muscles that can be targeted with a particular movement. This is feedback you don't get from fitness videos or at the gym, unless you have an experienced training partner or personal trainer.

Table 3-2	Master List of Strength-Training Exercises			
Exercise	*Target*	*Purpose*	*Menu Row*	*Advanced User?**
Single-Leg Extension	Triceps, Torso, and Hips	Tone and Coordination	First	No
Push-Up and Side Plank	Chest, Shoulders, and Arms	Tone	First	No

(continued)

Table 3-2 *(continued)*

Exercise	Target	Purpose	Menu Row	Advanced User?*
Torso Twist	Side Abdominals	Tone	First	No
Jackknife	Abdominals	Tone	First	No
Lunge	Thighs and Hips	Tone	First	No
Rowing Squat	Thighs and Back	Tone and Posture	Second	No
Single-Leg Twist	Side Abdominals	Tone	Second	No
Sideways Leg Lift	Side Abdominals and Shoulders	Tone	Second	No
Plank	Core	Flexibility and Posture	Second	No
Tricep Extension	Triceps	Tone	Second	No
Arm and Leg Lift	Shoulders and Hips	Tone and Balance	Third	Yes
Single-Arm Stand	Abdominals and Thighs	Tone and Coordination	Third	Yes
Balance Bridge	Triceps, Core, Buttocks	Tone and Balance	Third	Yes
Side Lunge	Rib Muscles (Intercostals) and Inner Thighs	Tone and Flexibility	Third	Yes
Single Leg Reach	Thighs, Buttocks, and Core	Tone and Balance	Third	Yes
Push-Up Challenge	Chest, Shoulders, and Arms	Tone	Fourth	No
Jackknife Challenge	Abdominals	Tone	Fourth	No
Plank Challenge	Core	Flexibility and Posture	Fourth	No

*Advanced User activities are those deemed to be more challenging by Wii Fit Plus.

Working your lower body

Whether you're walking about town or running up stairs, your legs are your base of power. Because your legs contain some of the largest muscle groups in your body, building these muscles gives you a leg up on your overall fat-burning efforts. Luckily, your leg muscles are also among the quickest to respond to training, so they will be among the first areas where you can achieve visible results.

Single-Leg Extension

Like most of the *Wii Fit Plus* strength-training movements, the Single-Leg Extension does not fit neatly into one body part category or section. In this case, the Single-Leg Extension is a compound movement that involves the back of the arm (triceps), the abs, and the front (quads) and bottom (calf) of the leg, requiring a good deal of coordination and balance. Perform the exercise by following these steps:

1. **Start with both feet on the Balance Board, and then lift and stretch your right leg backward as you move your right arm upward and forward.**

   Your left leg is used for balance and support, so it helps to tense your quads and calf throughout the set, as well as your abs.

   At the top of the movement, your right leg, torso, and right arm should be in a straight line at a roughly 45-degree angle.

2. **As you fully extend your right arm, flex your triceps to maximize impact on the muscle. Similarly, as you fully extend your right leg, flex your buttocks.**

3. **As you return to the starting position, your right foot remains raised to roughly just below the top of your left calf muscle rather than back on the Balance Board.**

4. **Repeat the motion for the indicated number of repetitions before placing both feet back on the Balance Board and performing the same movement with the other side of your body.**

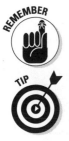

You must proactively maintain your balance by keeping the red dot on the screen within the yellow balance zone.

Performing strength-training exercises at a fast pace places a high level of stress on the muscles and connective tissue at the beginning of each movement. Performing them at a slower pace requires a more even application of muscle force throughout the movement range and produces greater muscle tension. Although *Wii Fit Plus* helps you regulate speed for many exercises, another great way to add further challenge to your exercise regimen is simply to slow down.

Lunge

Lunges are not just for fencers, they're also a great way for the rest of us to work our upper legs and buttocks. Though *Wii Fit Plus* suggests that the lunge is good for toning — which we are not denying — it is also a test of balance. Follow these steps:

1. **Start by clasping your hands behind your head and maintaining a rigid posture, with your chin up and your eyes looking straight ahead.**

   Keep your abs tensed the whole time to help maintain this posture.

2. **Step onto the Balance Board, and then move your left leg back.**

   At this point, your left knee should be at a roughly 90-degree angle and directly above your toes.

3. **Slowly descend until your left knee is nearly touching the ground, and the onscreen progress bar passes the indicator line.**

4. **While maintaining your posture, drive your body upward.**

5. **Repeat for the required number of repetitions before performing the same movement with your right leg.**

Rowing Squat

The squat is often called the "King of Exercises" and with good reason. Besides being extremely challenging, it's one of the most powerful ways to build strength and muscle in your upper thighs and buttocks. *Wii Fit Plus* incorporates a variation on the traditional squat by incorporating a rowing motion that involves the back muscles. Although your body weight provides sufficient resistance when squatting, the effect on the back when rowing is purely from how you contract and squeeze those muscles. Follow these steps:

1. **Start by placing both feet on the Balance Board and then placing both arms straight out in front of you, palms facing down.**

   Keep your head up and your stomach muscles contracted the whole time.

2. **As you slowly bend your knees, start to pull your arms down and back to just above your belly button until your palms face each other at the side of your body, contracting and squeezing your back muscles.**

   If done correctly, your back muscles should be at maximum contraction while you're at the low point of the squat. As indicated by the red dot on the screen, try to keep your center of balance in the blue area.

3. **Reverse the motion to return to the starting position and complete your first rep.**

4. **Continue the movement for the indicated number of repetitions.**

You can make the rowing squat more challenging by squatting even lower. Just be sure to maintain your center of balance at all times.

Single-Arm Stand

The Single-Arm Stand, which targets your abdominals and thighs, is an exercise that requires a great deal of coordination. Follow these steps:

1. **Start by lying on your back with your left arm fully extended and holding the Wii Remote.**

2. **With your left arm still extended, use your right arm to begin to push your body up while keeping your abs tensed.**

3. **Complete the movement by standing fully upright, continuing to keep your left arm fully extended and legs tensed.**

   The onscreen red line monitors your balance throughout the movement.

4. **Continue performing the Single-Arm Stand for the required number of reps, and then repeat for the other side.**

Side Lunge

Side Lunges target the major muscles of the lower body, but may place less strain on your knees. *Wii Fit Plus* adds a stretch to this activity, allowing you to work the muscles between your ribs (intercostals) simultaneously. Perform the activity by following these steps:

1. **Stand on the Balance Board and extend your left leg out to the side, about the distance of one Wii Balance Board.**

2. **Extend your left arm upward and place your right hand across your left side so that it rests on your stomach at roughly your navel.**

3. **Bend your right leg and lean over your right side, as shown in Figure 3-5.**

   Stabilize your balance in your bent leg as you stretch. Be careful not to let the knee of your bent leg extend past your toes.

4. **Return to the start position and repeat the motions for the required number of repetitions. Repeat for the other side.**

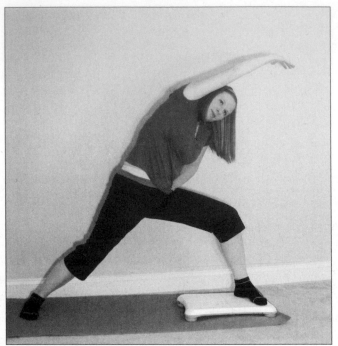

Figure 3-5:
Side Lunge
apex.

Single-Leg Reach

The Single-Leg Reach targets your thighs, buttocks, and core, while putting your balancing abilities to the test. This activity is advanced, so you may want to enlist the help of a spotter on your first attempt while following these steps:

1. **Stand on the Balance Board and slowly move your left hand and left leg simultaneously.**

   Your left hand will be above your head and your knee will be bent and raised so that your upper leg is parallel to the floor.

2. **Bring your left leg back, lower your left hand down to the floor, and hold this position, as shown in Figure 3-6.**

   Your upper body should be parallel to the floor.

3. **Lift your body back up and repeat for the required number of repetitions. Once complete, repeat for the other side.**

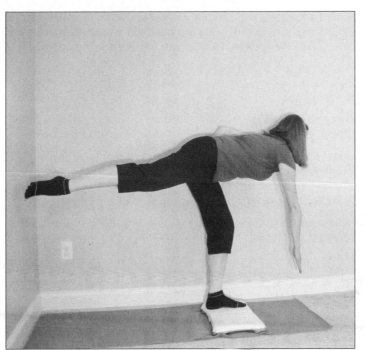

Figure 3-6:
Single-Leg
Reach apex.

Working your upper body

If you consider all your daily activities, you may find that most require use of your upper body. Many of these activities aren't given a second thought, such as opening a door — unless, of course, a particularly heavy one is encountered. By regularly working your upper body, many daily activities will become much easier, and there will be fewer doors you can't open. While gaining definition in your upper body may take longer to achieve, you don't need 20-inch biceps to be strong; even spaghetti arms can be powerful. Of course for many, the muscles of the upper body are considered the "show muscles," so aesthetics alone may be reason enough to work the area hard.

Push-Up and Side Plank

The Push-Up and Side Plank is another example of *Wii Fit Plus* taking a relatively straightforward movement — the push-up (also known as press-up) — and adding an additional step that ratchets up the difficulty, in this case the side plank. Push-ups work the pectoral (chest) muscles and arms, and side planks tone the shoulders and arms. Follow these steps:

1. **Start by placing your hands an equal distance apart on the Balance Board and extending your legs behind you until your entire body is in the raised and prone position on the balls of your feet.**

   It is important to stabilize your entire body before proceeding from this step so that you can maintain your form and balance throughout the movement.

2. **Once stabilized, follow *Wii Fit Plus*'s prompts to bend just your arms down, then back up, where you should squeeze your chest.**

3. **Once at the top position and prompted to do so, move to the Side Plank by extending your right arm off the Balance Board and back while your right leg moves behind your left foot, as shown in Figure 3-7. On full arm extension, squeeze your right triceps.**

4. **When prompted, move your right leg and right arm back to their original positions.**

   For the next rep, repeat the same sequence for the other side of your body.

The closer together your hands are when performing push-ups, the less you emphasize your chest and the more you emphasize your triceps.

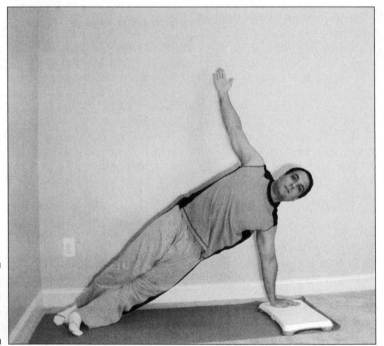

Figure 3-7:
Push-Up and Side Plank apex.

Plank

In some countries, the Plank is called a parallel stretch, and with good reason, as it's a literal description of the exercise. The Plank helps to strengthen your core muscles, including your abdominals, which can increase flexibility and improve posture. Follow these steps to do the Plank:

1. **Start by placing your forearms on the Balance Board and loosely grip the end with your fingers.**

2. **Extend your legs out and rise up on the balls of your feet as if you're about to do a push-up, but leave your arms in place.**

3. **Use your abdominals and other core muscles to stabilize and hold your position while keeping your balance to hold the onscreen dot as steady as possible for the predetermined length of time.**

Tricep Extension

You can put your Balance Board aside for this one, because all you need is the Wii Remote. As you might guess, Tricep Extensions work your triceps (the back muscles of your upper arms). Follow these steps:

1. **Grasp the Wii Remote in your left hand and raise your arm so it's pointing straight up, parallel to your head. Use your right hand to stabilize the back of your left arm just below the elbow.**

2. **Follow the onscreen indicator and extend your left arm, being sure to squeeze the triceps when you reach the top.**

3. **After completing the required number of repetitions, repeat for the other arm.**

Arm and Leg Lift

The Arm and Leg Lift is another one of those exercise combinations that defies easy categorization and is equally at home under Lower Body, because it works your upper leg and buttocks. However, it is listed here under Upper Body, because it also works your triceps and shoulders. Like the Tricep Extension, the Arm and Leg Lift is performed with just the Wii Remote. Follow these steps:

1. **Start in a stabilized kneeling position on all fours with the Wii Remote in your left hand.**

2. **Extend your left arm and right leg at the first whistle, squeezing your triceps and buttocks at full extension.**

3. **Using the onscreen guide, hold this position steady until the second whistle, at which time you return your left arm and right leg to the starting position.**

4. **Perform the required number of repetitions, and then repeat for the other side.**

Balance Bridge

The Balance Bridge works your triceps, core, and buttocks. Although you will be on the ground for this activity, a great deal of balance is required, as the name of this exercise implies. This exercise is an advanced activity, and you may want to enlist the help of a spotter before following these steps:

1. **Sit on the Balance Board, place your hands behind you for support, and bend your legs in front of you.**

   Make sure your body is fully supported before you proceed.

2. **Lift your hips and straighten your arms while extending your right leg when the Raise triangle aligns with the yellow triangle at the top meter.**

   Keep your upper body aligned with your lower body, so that it appears that you are forming a bridge, as shown in Figure 3-8. Your back should be straight and parallel to the ground.

3. **Bring your buttocks down and leg back in after the yellow triangle clears the Raise bar, and repeat the entire sequence for the required number of repetitions.**

4. **Repeat for the other leg.**

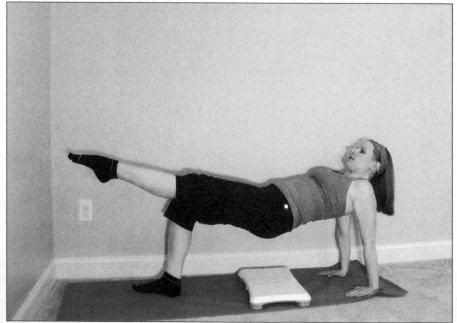

Figure 3-8:
Balance
Bridge apex.

Whittling your waistline

Washboard abs certainly rank high (if not highest) on most people's wish list. The good news is that unlike other body parts, it is difficult to overtrain your abs, since they recover from exercise stress quickly. Because you want to keep your abs tensed when doing all the other exercises, you'll be working them constantly; however, *Wii Fit Plus* has strength-training moves that specifically target this often problem area.

Abdominal exercises alone will not reduce the waist or define this muscle group. Only in conjunction with a healthy diet and a drop in body fat will you be able to see a change in definition.

Torso Twists

If you have "love handles" that you do not love, this exercise is for you! Torso Twists are especially effective at targeting the side abdominal muscles. To chisel your abdomen, follow these steps:

1. **Start with your feet shoulder-width apart on the Balance Board with your toes pointed slightly out.**

2. **Raise your arms to the side so that they are shoulder height and your palms are facing down.**

   Make sure that you keep your core, especially your abs, tight at all times.

3. **Using controlled movements, twist your torso from left to right, slowly moving your left shoulder forward and down as you twist so that your left arm is pointing down and your right arm is elevated above your head.**

   Your arms will end perpendicular to the Balance Board.

4. **Repeat this movement on the other side, twisting from right to left, for the required number of repetitions.**

Avoid moving your hips or bending your back. Twist slowly and within your limits to avoid injury.

Jackknife

What is the first exercise that pops into your head when you think of working your abdomen? We would wager it is the sit-up, which is precisely what the Jackknife improves upon. Follow these steps:

1. **Start by lying on the floor with your knees bent, heels resting on the Balance Board with your toes pointed up at an approximately 45-degree angle, and arms stretched out above your head.**

2. **At the sound of the first whistle, raise your legs and upper body at the same time, so that you form a V shape.**

3. **At the second whistle, lower your body to the start position. Squeeze and contract your abs as you lift your body.**

4. **Perform the required number of repetitions.**

   Do this exercise slowly; too much momentum can cause you to strain your back.

Single-Leg Twist

This exercise is another to add to your muffin-top-fighting arsenal. Single-leg twists target the oblique muscles, or sides, of your waistline. Follow these steps:

1. **Place your right hand on your hip, raise your left hand above your head, and lift your right leg off the Balance Board, making sure there is a slight bend in your knee.**

2. **Simultaneously raise your right leg and lower your left arm, bringing your right knee and left hand together at roughly your midline, as shown in Figure 3-9.**

3. **Bring your arm and leg back to the starting position. After your set, repeat on the other side.**

Because you are balancing yourself on one leg throughout this exercise, watch your posture to make sure that you stabilize your upper body to keep from leaning forward.

Sideways Leg Lift

Unlike the other *Wii Fit Plus* waistline moves, this one works your shoulders in addition to the side abdominal muscles, also known as the oblique muscles. Follow these steps:

1. **Start this exercise with your right hand on your right hip, then raise your left hand above your head while lifting your right leg sideways off the Balance Board.**

   Your right leg will be approximately at the height of the opposing knee and there should be no bend in either knee.

2. **Lower your right leg so that it hovers just above the Balance Board and is parallel to your left leg, while at the same time slowly bringing your left arm down enough for your fingers to be pointed toward the ground.**

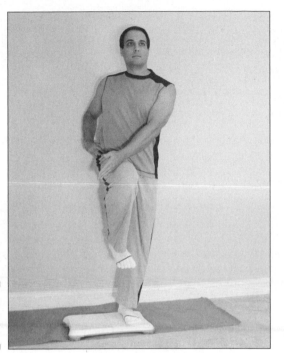

Figure 3-9:
Single-Leg
Twist apex.

3. **After you complete all your repetitions, repeat this movement on the opposite side.**

Keep your body steady as you move your arms and legs, and make sure to squeeze your shoulder muscles and your abs when you lift your arm and leg, respectively.

Stepping up to the challenges

If you do well in the higher difficulty settings of the Push-Up and Side Plank, Jackknife, and Plank, you will unlock these challenges, respectively, which appear in the fourth row of the Strength Training exercise selector menu. When performing challenges, your virtual trainer's personality changes from supportive to competitive, and you can put the proverbial metal to the virtual pedal and really test your limits. The goal is to outperform the virtual trainer in the number of repetitions performed or to hold a pose for longer.

Push-Up Challenge

Challenge your virtual trainer to see who can do more Push-ups. You do consecutive sets of ten repetitions at a time until either you or the trainer can't do any more. If you beat the virtual trainer, he or she comes back stronger the next time you try, increasing the challenge until you are able to reach 100 repetitions, at which point you will have maxed out on the challenge.

Listen to the whistle. It will be your guide for the correct Push-up timing. If your timing is off, it may not register as a repetition.

Plank Challenge

Unlike the other challenges, which are based on repetitions, the Plank Challenge tests who can hold the pose the longest. You do consecutive sets of ten seconds each until either you or the trainer can't do any more. If you beat the virtual trainer, he or she holds the Plank longer the next time you try, increasing the challenge until you're able to reach 180 seconds, at which point you'll have maxed out on the challenge.

Jackknife Challenge

You really feel the burn in your abs as you challenge your virtual trainer to see who can do more Jackknifes. You do consecutive sets of ten repetitions at a time until either you or the trainer can't do any more. If you beat the virtual trainer, he or she comes back stronger the next time you try, increasing the challenge until you're able to reach 100 repetitions, at which point you'll have maxed out on the challenge.

Chapter 4

Working Out with My Wii Fit Plus

....

....

*O*ne of the criticisms of the original *Wii Fit* was that it did not offer any routines. The *Wii Fit Plus* developers address such criticism through My Wii Fit Plus. You can choose from a list of routines that are designed to help you achieve a certain goal, such as youth or health, or you can try your hand at designing your own routine. If you like elements of two different routines, *Wii Fit Plus* even lets you combine them; the options are virtually limitless. Certainly, having so many choices helps prevent boredom and keeps you engaged.

In this chapter, we review all that My Wii Fit Plus has to offer, including how to build your own routines and combine routines. We also provide a table of the preset routines for you to easily refer back to, and discuss some of the icons on the My Wii Fit Plus screen, such as the Calorie Check.

Starting My Wii Fit Plus

You can access My Wii Fit Plus from the Training Menu or by clicking on the door on the Calendar screen. The My Wii Fit Plus screen resembles a locker room, which is fitting considering that it serves as workout central when it comes to routines. You also encounter an old friend here, your virtual Balance Board. If you click on him, you can practice any of the ten available Balance Tests, provided you've done them before while taking a Body Test.

For more on the Balance Tests, turn to Chapter 2.

You have several options to choose from on the My Wii Fit Plus screen, including Calorie Check, Fit Credits, Change Trainer, and What are METs? icons on the left and Wii Fit Plus Routines, My Routine, and Favorites buttons on the right, as shown in Figure 4-1. The following sections help you discover what these options are all about.

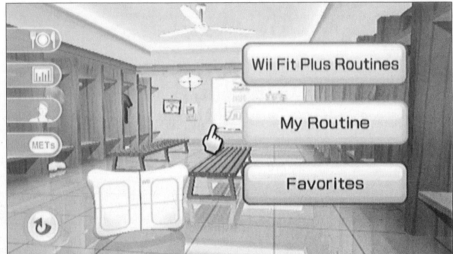

Figure 4-1:
My Wii Fit
Plus screen.

Going Over the Icons

Although it doesn't take a Sherlock Holmes to figure out what lies behind those four icons on the My Wii Fit Plus screen, our job is to ensure that you have all the information necessary to make the most of *Wii Fit Plus*. So, bear with us as we quickly walk you through what each of these icons has to offer.

Burning calories

Clicking on the Fork, Plate, and Knife icon allows you to set the number of calories you'd like to burn daily by clicking on the Calorie Burn Goal button. You can use this feature to see how many calories you need to burn to counter that hot-fudge sundae you've just eaten. Follow these steps to set your Calorie Burn Goal:

1. **Browse through the food items, as shown in Figure 4-2, for informational purposes or if you want to find the calorie count for a food you wish to burn off.**

2. **When you are ready to set your caloric goal, click the green Calorie Burn Goal button at the bottom right of the screen.**

   Doing this pulls up the Goal Food menu, as shown in Figure 4-3.

3. **From this menu, select the food item that represents the number of calories you want to burn daily.**

   As you hover over the Goal Food items, you can see how many calories they have.

4. **When you are happy with your selection, click the Set button or click the Back button if you prefer to select a different Goal Food item.**

   Keep in mind that you can change this goal anytime by clicking on Calorie Burn Goal and selecting Remove or Change. Remove erases your daily goal settings, whereas Change pulls up the Goal Food menu again. Simply click on the item you want, and your new goal is set.

The highest Goal Food item is a chocolate bar at 455 calories, whereas the scroll-through list includes food items up to a calorie count of 860. Although you can't set your Calorie Burn Goal that high, you gain a good perspective on how many calories foods you may regularly eat or drink contain. For example, you may think that the taco salad you like to eat for lunch is a healthy option, only to discover that it actually has a whopping 655 calories. You can use this feature as a nutritional guide, and if there are items not on the list that you are curious about, you can visit the same source from where this information came: USDA National Nutrient Database for Standard Reference. You can access it by visiting www.nal.usda.gov/fnic/foodcomp/search.

After you finish your workout, you can check how close you are to your Calorie Burn Goal by clicking on the Fork, Plate, and Knife icon. Your calories burned for that day are displayed in red on top of the scroll-through list. You can also see how many calories are left to reach your goal after you complete a workout through Wii Fit Plus Routines.

Checking Fit Credits

Clicking on the Graph icon enables you to check how many Fit Credits are in your Fit Bank, and they are color coded so that you see how your Fit Credits were earned. The default is a 1-week view, but you can see larger time intervals by clicking the + and – signs onscreen or on your Wii Remote.

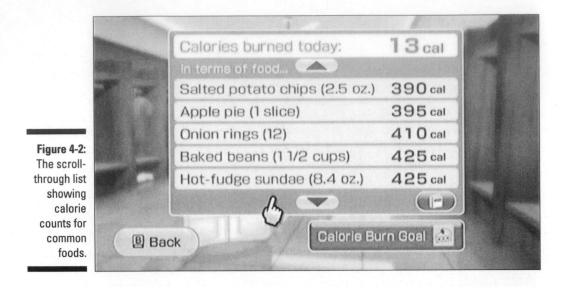

Figure 4-2:
The scroll-through list showing calorie counts for common foods.

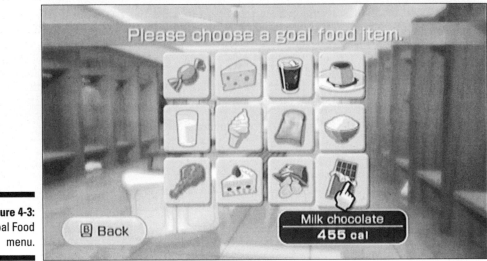

Figure 4-3:
Goal Food menu.

Changing your trainer

Clicking on the Face icon enables you to change between the male and female trainer. After you select a trainer, you are asked if that is the trainer you want. If so, click OK, and if not, click the Back button to choose the one you really meant. Consider switching trainers every few workouts to help mix things up. To keep things interesting, the trainers' hairstyles change every so often, and one day you may find your male trainer sporting a new ponytail.

Understanding METs

This icon is available only after you've spent some time training with *Wii Fit Plus* and have already been presented with a definition of METs, which are metabolic equivalents of task. You can turn to Chapter 1 for more on METs. We've also included tables in Chapters 3, 5, and 6 that list the MET value for each activity discussed in those chapters. When the MET icon becomes available to you in My Wii Fit Plus, you can click on it anytime to get a recap of METs and calorie expenditure.

Working Out with Wii Fit Plus Routines

The *Wii Fit Plus* routines are designed to help you target certain areas, such as a specific body part or your balance skills. You can select from Lifestyle, Health, Youth, and Form, each of which has three different focus areas with its own routines, all of which include three exercises, as shown in Table 4-1. You can opt to perform only one of the routines from these focus areas by clicking the one you want and then selecting Start. You can also opt to create your own routine by combining the available routines, which can be done by clicking the Combine button at the Wii Fit Plus Routines Menu screen. Whereas My Routines only allows you to select Yoga and Strength Training activities, these incorporate other *Wii Fit Plus* activities.

Table 4-1	Master List of Wii Fit Plus Routines		
Workout Title	*Activities*	*Objective*	*Approximate Workout Time*
Lifestyle			
Shoulders and back	Torso Twists, Palm Tree, and Big Top Juggling	Relax shoulders and lower back	6 minutes
Relax	Deep Breathing, Sun Salutation, and Rhythm Parade	Calm and relax	7 minutes
Warm up	Warrior, Bird's Eye Bull's Eye, Downward-Facing Dog	Get blood flowing	6 minutes

(continued)

Table 4-1 *(continued)*

Workout Title	Activities	Objective	Approximate Workout Time
Health			
Tummy	Jackknife, Single-Leg Twist, and Snowball Fight	Burn fat around waistline	5 minutes
Overindulged	Basic Run, Rhythm Boxing, and Lunge	Burn unwanted calories	8 minutes
Leaner Mii	Hula Hoop, Island Cycling, and Skateboard Arena	Burn unwanted fat	8 minutes
Youth			
Posture	Tree, Half-Moon, and Lotus Focus	Improve posture and sense of overall well-being	6 minutes
Mind and body	Perfect 10, Table Tilt, and Obstacle Course	Improve mind and body coordination	7 minutes
Legs and hips	Step Basics, Chair, and Rowing Squat	Strengthen legs and hips	6 minutes
Form			
Hips	Single-Leg Extension, Advance Step, and Standing Knee	Improve posture	8 minutes
Arms	Rhythm Kung Fu, Tricep Extension, and Balance Bridge	Tone upper arms	6 minutes
Figure	Hula Hoop, Sideways Leg Lift, and Triangle	Shape figure	7 minutes

Combining routines

After you click the Combine button at the Wii Fit Plus Routines Menu screen, a menu appears with icons representing the 12 workout options offered through Wii Fit Plus Routines, as shown in Figure 4-4. The icons are color coded by category, with blue for Lifestyle, yellow for Health, green for Youth, and pink for Form. Hovering over each icon gives you the workout title. Refer to Table 4-1 for the activities included under each workout title. You can also choose from three activity levels, including one at a time, two at a time, and three at a time. Selecting one at a time randomly pulls one exercise from each of the workouts you've selected, two at a time randomly pulls two exercises, and three at a time includes all the exercises. Any routines you combine are one-time use and are not stored. If you want to perform the same activities again, you have to make the same selections, but there are no guarantees that the workout will be the same unless you choose three at a time. As you add activities, you can see the approximate workout time just above the Start button. You also cannot include a particular workout more than once on your exercise queue.

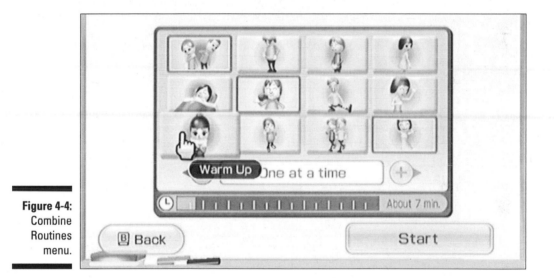

Figure 4-4:
Combine
Routines
menu.

Making My Routine

As the name implies, My Routine lets you to create your very own routine. Although *Wii Fit Plus* offers many different activities, the only ones available here are Yoga and Strength Training. This may be a bit of a disappointment, but Yoga and Strength Training exercises are the ones that whip you into shape, and you can always perform some of the other activities afterwards to reward yourself.

Creating your routine

After you click on My Routine, you see Yoga and Strength tabs at the top, as shown in Figure 4-5. You can toggle between them to select the exercises you want by pointing to the desired exercise and then pressing A. After you have chosen an exercise, a yellow frame appears around it, and you see it listed on the right in the Selected Exercises menu. Unlike in My Wii Fit Plus Routines, you can select the same exercise more than once. To swap exercises, point to the one you wish to eliminate from your repertoire and press A, and then click on its replacement and press A again. To remove an exercise from your routine, press B. If you want to start from scratch, click the dial-like button to the left of the Start button, which resets the workout. Be careful. After you click this button, your items are instantly deleted. As you add or remove items, you can see the total workout time listed directly above the Start button increase or decrease, respectively. When you are happy with your workout, click the Start button to begin. Table 4-2 is a master list of exercises that indicate whether they target your upper or lower body and if they are good for warming up and cooling down. You can refer to this table to customize your routine, and whether you want to target your upper body, lower body, or entire body.

Table 4-2	Master Exercise List for Creating Your Routines		
Exercise	*Upper Body*	*Lower Body*	*Warm Up/Cool Down*
Yoga			
Deep Breathing	No	No	Yes
Half-Moon	No	No	Yes
Warrior	No	Yes	Yes
Tree	Yes	Yes	No
Sun Salutation	Yes	Yes	No
Standing Knee	No	Yes	No
Palm Tree	Yes	Yes	No
Chair	Yes	Yes	No
Triangle	Yes	Yes	No
Downward-Facing Dog	Yes	No	Yes
Dance	Yes	Yes	No

Exercise	Upper Body	Lower Body	Warm Up/Cool Down
Cobra	Yes	No	No
Bridge	No	Yes	No
Spinal Twist	Yes	No	No
Shoulder Stand	Yes	No	No
Spine Extension	Yes	Yes	No
Gate	Yes	Yes	No
Grounded V	Yes	No	No
Strength			
Single-Leg Extension	No	Yes	No
Push-Up and Side Plank	Yes	No	Yes
Torso Twist	Yes	No	No
Jackknife	Yes	No	No
Lunge	No	Yes	No
Rowing Squat	Yes	No	No
Single-Leg Twist	Yes	No	Yes
Sideways Leg Lift	Yes	No	Yes
Plank	Yes	No	Yes
Tricep Extension	Yes	No	Yes
Arm and Leg Lift	Yes	Yes	Yes
Single-Arm Stand	Yes	No	No
Balance Bridge	Yes	Yes	No
Side Lunge	No	Yes	No
Single Leg Reach	No	Yes	No

Wondering what the virtual Wii Balance Board is up to? If you click on it, it will create a routine for you based on how much time you have available and which exercises you want to incorporate, as shown in Figure 4-6. You can select from 5 minutes up to 60 minutes by clicking on the + and – buttons onscreen or on your Wii Remote. Select Yoga to include only yoga poses in your workout. Select Strength if you prefer only strength training activities. You can also select both to create a workout with a combination of the two. The activities that will be included in your workout are listed on the right.

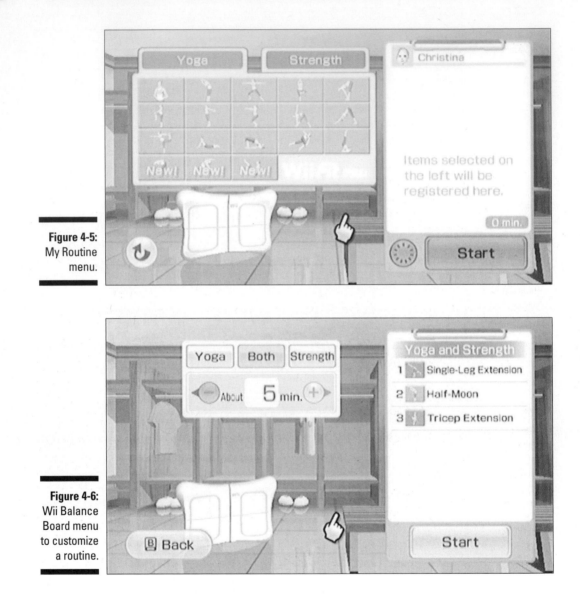

Figure 4-5:
My Routine
menu.

Figure 4-6:
Wii Balance
Board menu
to customize
a routine.

Favorites

Clicking on Favorites on the My Wii Fit Plus screen pulls up a menu that shows the ten exercises you've done most frequently, recently, and rarely, as shown in Figure 4-7. Although you can see how many times you've performed an exercise when you click on an activity from any exercise selector menu accessed through the Training Menu, having a ranked list can be helpful. After all, human being are creatures of habit and there are certain activities that we naturally gravitate to, often without even thinking about it. These lists can help you keep challenging yourself by showing you trends, which may serve as the impetus to move you out of your comfort zone. For example, you can see if you frequently perform activities focused mostly on one body part or whether you perform one type of activity, such as strength training. If so, you can customize your workouts to address this, or simply pick some of your rarely performed activities and put those into your next workout.

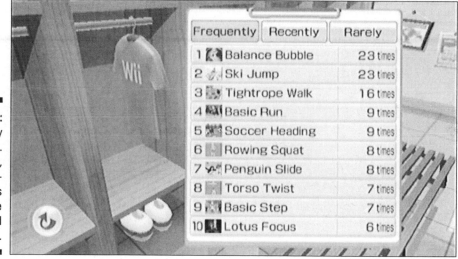

Figure 4-7:
Frequently
menu.
Clearly,
some-
one likes
Balance
Bubble and
Ski Jump.

Chapter 5

Breaking a Sweat with Aerobics

Many people equate exercising with performing aerobic activities, such as running on a treadmill or bicycling, because there are more immediate effects: Your heart starts pounding, sweat starts dripping, and your body starts to feel the burn, psychologically indicating fat is melting away. Although aerobic exercises shouldn't be your sole form of exercise, they are an extremely important component of a well-rounded physical fitness regimen. Aerobic activities improve the efficiency of your heart, lungs, and circulatory system when performed regularly.

Wii Fit Plus's aerobic exercises meet all the criteria for a good aerobic workout, but unlike riding a stationary bike or walking a treadmill, these activities also keep you mentally engaged, whether by catching hoops or looking for hidden *Super Mario Bros.* icons on the jogging trails.

In this chapter, you are introduced to the various *Wii Fit Plus* aerobic exercises, including descriptions of each one. Tips on performing the exercises are also provided.

Getting Started

To access the aerobics exercises, select the red Aerobics button on the Training menu. Once at the Aerobics Selector Menu, pick the activity you want to perform. Table 5-1 outlines the available *Wii Fit Plus* aerobics activities, including those that appear under Training Plus, which is covered in Chapter 6. After you select an activity, you see the game summary information, including which equipment is needed for the activity and how many metabolic equivalent of tasks (METs) the activity is worth, and you have the choice of two options: Back and Start. Selecting Back takes you back to the Aerobics Selector Menu. Selecting Start will proceed directly into training at the Activity Level indicated; the Hula Hoop, Basic Step, and Advanced Step have only one Activity Level. If an exercise has additional Activity Levels that have been unlocked, these can be accessed by clicking the + on your Wii Remote. Click – on the screen or the Wii Remote to go to a lower Activity Level.

Any time during the activity, you can press + on the Wii Remote to access the pause menu, which will give you the option to continue playing the current session, retry the activity (this restarts the activity), or quit the activity and return to the Aerobics Selector Menu.

Table 5-1	Master List of Aerobics Exercises*	
Activity	*MET Value*	*Equipment Needed*
Running		
Basic Run	5.0	Wii Remote
2-P Run	5.0	Two Wii Remotes
Free Run	5.0	Wii Remote
Step Exercises		
Basic Step	3.0	Balance Board
Advanced Step	3.5	Balance Board
Free Step	3.0	Balance Board
Boxing		
Rhythm Boxing	3.5	Nunchuk, Wii Remote, Balance Board
Hula Hoop		
Hula Hoop	4.0	Balance Board
Super Hula Hoop	4.0	Balance Board
Training Plus		
Rhythm Kung Fu	3.0	Nunchuk, Wii Remote, Balance Board
Rhythm Parade	3.0	Nunchuk, Wii Remote, Balance Board
Basic Run Plus	4.0	Wii Remote

Toning Your Body

Wii Fit Plus offers nine aerobic exercises under the Aerobics Selector Menu, but four distinct activities: running, step exercises, boxing, and Hula Hoop, as outlined in Table 5-1. Running and step exercises are especially good at working the lower body, the Hula Hoop works your core muscles — your torso minus your arms and legs — and boxing trains your upper body; thus, all your major muscle groups are covered. Some additional aerobic exercises are offered under the Training Plus Selector Menu, including Rhythm Kung Fu, Rhythm Parade, and Basic Run Plus, and these options are described in detail in Chapter 6.

As you can see from Table 5-1, all of *Wii Fit Plus*'s aerobic activities are rated between 3.0 and 5.0 METs. Exercises between 3.0 and 6.0 METs are considered moderate-intensity physical activities, whereas those above 6.0 METs are considered vigorous physical activities. No activities in *Wii Fit Plus* are higher than 5 METs; thus, the intensity of your workouts is usually moderate. To reap the greatest benefit from these moderate-intensity aerobic activities, your target heart rate zone should be 50 to 75 percent of your maximum heart rate. Table 5-2 provides average target heart rates by age. See the "Determining target heart rate" sidebar for more on target heart rate.

Determining target heart rate

Monitoring your target heart rate is a simple way to assess your exercise intensity and track your fitness levels. All you have to do is periodically take your pulse as you exercise and then stay within 50 to 75 percent of your maximum heart rate, which is considered your target heart rate. Since your heart rate will start to go down after stopping the activity, be sure to take your pulse within five seconds of stopping to ensure the greatest accuracy. Count your pulse for ten seconds and then take that number and multiply it by six. Voila, you now have your pulse rate.

Table 5-2 shows estimated target heart rates for different ages. You can use this as a guide to determine your target heart rate by using the values for the age closest to your own. If your age is not listed or you prefer more exact numbers, even though the difference will be but a few beats, you can determine your target heart rate with a simple calculation. First, determine your maximum age-related heart rate by subtracting your age from 220. Take this number and multiply it by 50 percent and then by 75 percent. You've now got your target heart rate zone. Here is an example for a 32-year-old:

$220 - 32 = 188$

50 percent level: $.50 \times 188 = 94$

75 percent level: $.75 \times 188 = 141$

Target Heart Rate Zone: 94–141 beats per minute

Before starting any activities, be sure to warm up. You can do this by performing a graduated, low-intensity aerobic exercise, such as walking in place for a few minutes. Some of the lower-intensity aerobic exercises in *Wii Fit Plus* also work well, such as Rhythm Parade. For more on warming up (and cooling down), turn to Chapter 1.

If you are taking medications, especially certain blood pressure medications, these values may not apply to you, as some drugs lower the maximum heart rate and thus the target heart rate zone. If you are on any medications, it is strongly advised that you speak with your physician before using target heart rate to gauge your exercise intensity.

Table 5-2	Average Target Heart Rates by Age	
Age, years	Target Heart Rate (50%–75%), beats per minute	Average Maximum Heart Rate (100%), beats per minute
20	100–150	200
25	98–146	195
30	95–142	190
35	93–138	185
40	90–135	180
45	88–131	175
50	85–127	170
55	83–123	165
60	80–120	160
65	78–116	155
70	75–113	150

Pounding the pavement

Wii Fit Plus running activities (Basic Run, 2-P Run, and Free Run) are best performed by jogging in place at a steady pace. If you try running and end up going too fast, your Mii will fall and you will receive fewer Fit Credits at the end of the activity. Jogging is also less taxing on your body, especially if you are not used to running, and it allows you to increase your fitness levels. These activities are not performed on the Balance Board, so if you are going to be doing them on a hard surface (non-carpeted area), you may want to put on a pair of sneakers to minimize shock to your knees as you pound the proverbial pavement.

In addition to using *Wii Fit Plus* to track your progress, consider investing in a pedometer to see how many steps you are taking during these activities and daily. You may be surprised to find that you are not taking as many as you thought. Strive for 10,000 steps daily, which is equivalent to roughly 5 miles.

Basic Run

For this exercise, you are putting your Balance Board aside and your movements will be tracked by the Wii Remote. Place the Wii Remote in your pocket or hold onto it if you don't have pockets. If you hold onto the Wii Remote, make sure to use and secure the wrist strap to prevent the Wii Remote from dropping during the activity. After the countdown and Start prompt, begin jogging in place at a steady pace so that you won't pass the Mii guide in front of you. Your Mii guide is a generic Mii and not one on your system, though you will encounter familiar Miis along the way as you make your way through the course. Be sure not to go too fast; otherwise your Mii will end up falling. To optimize the calorie burning potential of this exercise, swing your arms in big motions as you jog; if you are holding the Wii Remote in your hands, your Mii may run faster if you swing your arms faster than the pace of your feet. Your advancement through the course is tracked by the meter at the bottom of the screen, along which a mini version of your Mii's head advances as you progress toward the goal. The medium-sized circle in the middle of the meter indicates the half-way point of the course, and *Wii Fit Plus* also alerts you when you have reached this point and provides encouragement to keep going.

Although your Mii will traverse picturesque island terrain on the Short Course, which is available from the outset, you would likely become bored if this course were your only option. Fortunately, there are numerous other courses that can be taken. There are two longer courses, the Long Course and the Island Lap Course, both of which need to be unlocked. The Long Course becomes available once the Short Course has been completed, and the Island Course becomes available once the Long Course has been completed. The trail options don't stop here though. On each of these courses, you can take an alternate course by following any of the single dogs that run past you — not those headed in a pack toward you. When you see one of these dogs, quickly run past your guide and start following the dog. An "Oh! You've passed your guide!" message appears, which is followed by "Now, follow the dog." If you see another single dog pass the one that you are following, you can elect to follow it instead, leading to yet more alternatives. To get an overview of the entire terrain and available trails, refer to the Wuhu Island Running Map in your *Wii Fit Plus* instruction booklet. In addition to taking in the various sites along the way, there are numerous iconic marks from *Super Mario Bros.* scattered about the island for you to discover, including Mario, Luigi, star men, magic mushrooms, and others; an example is shown in Figure 5-1. How many can you find?

The number of *Wii Fit Plus* credits achieved on each course varies based on your performance. A steady pace yields more credits than an erratic one, so the motto of "slow and steady wins the race" certainly goes a long way here.

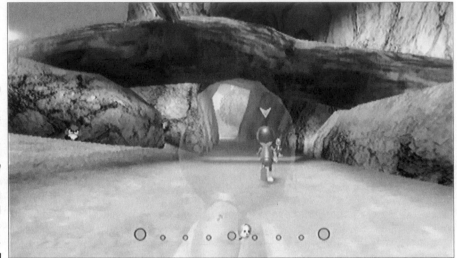

Figure 5-1:
One of the iconic marks from *Super Mario Bros.* on the Wuhu Island short trail during Basic Run.

2-P Run

This is the same as the Basic Run, except that you can now add a second player as a running partner. The screen is split for this activity. One side shows your Mii and the other your partner's generic Mii. As for all *Wii Fit Plus* running activities, your Balance Board is placed aside and you and your partner's movements are tracked by your respective Wii Remotes; however, only your results will be saved.

Free Run

For Free Run, you can run or jog in place for 10, 20, or 30 minutes. Initially, you are given ten minutes, but the other durations become available as you complete the subsequent activity. Although you can run the course on the screen, the idea of this mode is to allow you to watch TV while you work out. Verbal guidance is provided through the Wii Remote's speakers.

The prompts and feedback on your pace can be difficult to hear, especially if you have surround sound and are watching your favorite action movie. Increasing the volume of the Wii Remote in the Remote Setting menu may help; turn to Chapter 1 to find out how. It may also be best to hold the Wii Remote in your hand rather than putting it in your pocket, where the sound may become muffled by your clothes.

Stepping up to fitness

Step aerobics, which involves stepping up and down an elevated platform, originated in the late 1980s and quickly took off. Although this activity can provide a great workout, step bench heights generally range from four to ten inches, and the Balance Board has a height of just over two inches. As a result of this, you will not be working your muscles as intensely as you would with a traditional step aerobics program, and, therefore, won't reap as much physically from this activity as from some other *Wii Fit Plus* exercises.

If you find that you enjoy *Wii Fit Plus*'s step aerobics programs, you can consider purchasing a special riser to elevate your Balance Board to the standard 4-inch height, which gives a boost to the workout potential of this activity. Turn to Chapter 13 to find out more about this accessory.

Basic Step

This activity is the step aerobics take on *DanceDanceRevolution,* as you will be stepping on and off the Balance Board in a choreographed pattern based on the beat of the music and onscreen prompts, which consist of arrows and cute little feet that appear in a vertical scrolling panel in the middle of the screen. This panel resembles a series of Balance Boards, and when a board in this panel becomes yellow and is rimmed in red, it means you need to execute the move that is shown. The goal is to step on and off the board in sync with the other Miis, who happen to be master steppers and nod in appreciation at you when you are in step with them. Initially, the movements are quite basic, and you will simply be stepping up when you see the red feet and down when you see the red arrows. However, halfway through, things get more complicated with the introduction of blue feet and arrows, which requires you to step off to the side of the Balance Board. In some cases, a blue arrow and two feet on either side of a board in the scrolling panel appear, with one foot being a lighter blue, as shown in Figure 5-2. This light blue foot indicates the foot that stays put; only the darker foot moves per the prompt indicated. If you find these feet confusing, you can ignore them and just try to follow the blue arrows. The feet simply illustrate the foot placements that the blue directional arrows are indicating.

If following the onscreen prompts proves too challenging, try watching the Miis and following their movements until you get the hang of it and catch the beat.

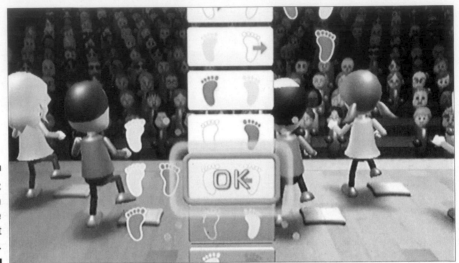

Figure 5-2:
A pattern
with the
blue feet
and arrows.

Advanced Step

This is a much faster version of the Basic Step with the introduction of two new moves. The activity starts the same as the Basic Step, with a set consisting of simply stepping on and off the board. Shortly thereafter, the side stepping with blue arrows and feet from Basic Step is introduced, except that you now also have to clap along with the other Miis when indicated, which you will be required to do for the remainder of the game; you will see little hand icons on the screen. Following a brief pause, a whole new move is introduced with green feet and arrows, which require you to kick your leg out in front of you; however, if you watch the Miis, they are not really kicking their legs out and are basically keeping their foot suspended in the air for the beat. After two rounds with the green feet and clapping, another new move is introduced with purple feet and arrows. You now have to step on and off the Balance Board sideways — first to the left and then to the right. Shortly thereafter, you go through the entire series of moves again, but at a much faster pace. As with Basic Step, if you have a tough time staying in sync with the beat, try following the Miis.

Free Step

If you want to step up and down on your Balance Board while watching your favorite television show, this is the activity for you. You can do this for 10, 20, or 30 minutes, though only 10 minutes is available to you initially. The Wii Remote speaker provides you with feedback and keeps you apprised of how much time you have left. It also plays a rhythmic tone for you to follow.

You can adjust the tempo of this tone by pressing up or down on the Wii Remote's directional pad. If you don't like the tone that is playing, you can change or eliminate it by pressing the A button. If you have a tough time hearing your Wii Remote speaker, you can adjust its volume by going into the Remote Settings menu; turn to Chapter 1 to find out how. You may also opt to hold the Wii Remote in your hand rather than putting it in your pocket, which may muffle the sound.

Knocking out fat

Punches have been thrown since the dawn of mankind, but the first historical records of boxing as a sport date back to the ancient Greeks. The sport has remained incredibly popular, with numerous styles developing through the ages in different cultures. Boxing has numerous benefits, especially when you do not have to worry about being pounded to a bloody pulp by an actual opponent. Some of these benefits include improved hand-eye coordination, increased strength and cardiovascular endurance, as well as improved fat burning. So put up your dukes and start throwing some punches, *Wii Fit Plus* style!

Rhythm Boxing

If you think you are going to have the opportunity to duke it out with another Mii, think again — this is family-friendly Nintendo, after all. Instead, you get to pound a punching bag with robot-like arms. Unlike all other activities, this game incorporates the Wii Remote, Balance Board, and Nunchuck. You are instructed to hold the Wii Remote in your right hand and the Nunchuck in the left, though you can switch hands at your discretion without penalty. Because this activity is not as straightforward as the other activities, it is essential to pay close attention as the Mii Trainer demonstrates each pattern of moves, which you have to mimic. To execute punches, you first have to step forward off the front of the Balance Board toward the punching bag. Your score is based on your timing, with each perfectly timed punch accruing two points versus one for less desirable moves. Try throwing punches immediately after the target appears on the punching bag. This activity has several durations, with three minutes being initially available. As the duration increases, so does the difficulty of the patterns that you must mimic. Toward the end of the three-minute exercise, there will be a five-second Bonus Time in which your trainer will allow you to throw punches any way you want to; see Figure 5-3. You do not have to step on and off the Balance Board for this round, so focus on racking up the points by getting in as many punches as possible to knock out your punching bag opponent. Longer durations have longer bonus rounds.

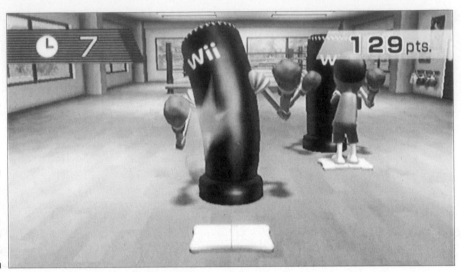

Figure 5-3:
The Rhythm
Boxing
bonus
round.

Getting your virtual hoop on

Although Hula Hoop is a registered trademark of Wham-O, Inc., a toy company that was founded in 1948 and is still in existence today, it is in fact an ancient invention that has been used throughout history by countless cultures for different purposes. It was also constructed of numerous materials, ranging from wood to grapevines. The plastic Hula Hoops that we know today were first commercialized in the late 1950s by Wham-O, and the craze quickly caught on, with over 100 million sold the first year it was on the market. More recently, use of hoops has emerged as an aerobic fitness trend, often referred to as *hooping* or *hoopdance,* though these activities tend to use custom, weighted hoops. Exercising with the Hula Hoop has numerous benefits beyond the cardiovascular, such as strengthening your core, increasing spinal flexibility, and improving coordination, all of which are also provided with *Wii Fit Plus*'s virtual hoop, so get those hips swaying.

Hula Hoop

The goal is to quickly rotate your hips in a circular motion to keep your Mii's Hula Hoop on its waist while getting in as many spins as possible in a 70-second period; the faster you spin, the more points you acquire. The timer appears at the top right of the screen and the spin meter appears at the top center of the screen. Two Miis holding Hula Hoops face you and will on occasion toss a Hula Hoop your Mii's way, which you have to catch, as shown by Figure 5-4. This can present quite a challenge. If you don't place enough weight on the proper side of the Balance Board to catch the Hula Hoop, your leaning won't register. One way to ensure you catch those Hula Hoops is to raise your arms above your head while leaning in the proper direction; this should be done immediately after the Hula Hoop is thrown. Once the Hula Hoop is caught, you should quickly get back into full swing to rack up as many points as possible, as each Hula Hoop caught will register as a rotation of your hips on the spin meter.

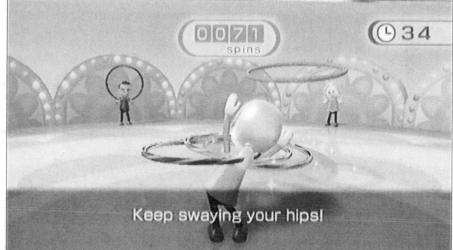

Figure 5-4:
A Hula Hoop being tossed with the Mii in position to catch it.

Keep swaying your hips!

Super Hula Hoop

The mechanics are the same as for Hula Hoop, except that there are two rounds, both of which put 180 seconds on the clock. For the first round, you sway your hips to the right, and for the second round, you sway them to the left. At the end of both of these rounds, *Wii Fit Plus* draws each of your rotations for each side on the screen and comes up with a schematic that illustrates your average rotation on the right and the left. It also indicates how many rotations were done on each side and proceeds to rank you.

Chapter 6

Training Plus and Balance Games

In this Chapter

▶ Getting started

▶ Discovering Training Plus games

▶ Targeting your vestibular system

▶ Exploring Balance Games

*K*eeping your muscles and cardiovascular system strong is important, but equally essential is honing your balance skills and keeping those mental muscles sharp. To facilitate this, *Wii Fit Plus* offers 24 game-based activities that test the reflexes, mind and body coordination, balance, and memory. Unlike other *Wii Fit Plus* activities, most of the Training Plus and Balance Games activities won't cause you to break a sweat, but they can be enjoyed by the whole family, including young children.

This chapter gives you an overview of all *Wii Fit Plus* Training Plus and Balance Games activities, reviewing game mechanics and scoring. Screenshots are provided for select activities. The role of the vestibular system in achieving balance is also discussed. Because these games are all quite gentle, requiring subtle movements, or in the case of the meditative Lotus Focus (a Balance Game), extreme focus while sitting motionless on the Balance Board, they can be used as part of the warm-up regimen before starting any of the other *Wii Fit Plus* activities. See Chapter 1 for more on warming up. They also can be used to test your mastery of some of the other *Wii Fit Plus* activities that require you to balance yourself, such as the one-legged yoga poses that are discussed in Chapter 3.

Starting Training Plus and Balance Games

To access the Training Plus activities, select the gray Training Plus button on the Training menu, or to get to the Balance Games, click the yellow Balance Games button instead. At the Training Plus or Balance Games selector menu,

_____

pick the activity you want to perform. After you select an activity, you see the game summary information, including which equipment is needed for the activity and how many metabolic equivalent of tasks (METs) the activity is worth. You have the choice of two options: Back and Start. Selecting Back takes you back to the Training Plus or Balance Games selector menu, depending upon which one you were on. Selecting Start proceeds directly into training at the activity level indicated. If you've already unlocked additional activity levels on a particular game, these can be accessed by clicking the + on the screen or pressing the + on the Wii Remote. Click − on the screen or press − on the Wii Remote to go to a lower activity level.

You can press + on the Wii Remote any time during a game to access the pause menu, which gives you the option to Continue Playing the Current Session, Retry to restart the activity, or to Quit, which brings you back to the Training Plus or Balance Games selector menu.

Exploring Training Plus

All training options listed under the Training menu are self-explanatory, except, perhaps, Training Plus. This option is new to *Wii Fit Plus* and features 15 assorted activities, as shown in Figure 6-1, including some balance games, aerobic activities, agility tests, and exercises that engage the mind. Table 6-1 is a master list of Training Plus activities and their objectives. Because this option is unique to *Wii Fit Plus,* even *Wii Fit* gurus may want an overview of this uncharted territory.

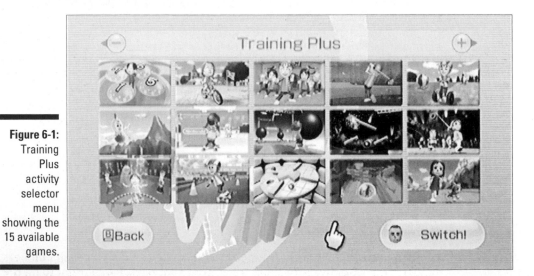

Figure 6-1: Training Plus activity selector menu showing the 15 available games.

Table 6-1	Master List of Training Plus Games		
Game	*METs Burned*	*Equipment*	*Objective*
Perfect 10	2.5	Balance Board	Tests your body and mind coordination
Island Cycling	2.5	Balance Board, Wii Remote	Works your lower body
Rhythm Kung Fu	3.0	Balance Board, Wii Remote, Nunchuk	Tests your sense of rhythm and coordination
Driving Range	3.0	Balance Board, Wii Remote	Analyzes your golf swing
Segway Circuit	2.0	Balance Board, Wii Remote	Tests your balance and agility
Bird's-Eye Bull's Eye	2.5	Balance Board	Tests your upper body strength and sense of balance
Snowball Fight	2.0	Balance Board, Wii Remote	Trains your judgment skills and reaction time
Obstacle Course	3.0	Balance Board	Tests your timing and agility
Tilt City	2.0	Balance Board, Wii Remote	Tests your hand-eye coordination
Rhythm Parade	3.0	Balance Board, Wii Remote, Nunchuk	Trains your sense of rhythm and coordination
Big Top Juggling	2.0	Balance Board, Wii Remote, Nunchuk	Tests your sense of balance and timing
Skateboard Arena	3.0	Balance Board	Tests your balance and agility
Table Tilt Plus	1.5	Balance Board	Tests your overall balance and coordination
Balance Bubble Plus	2.0	Balance Board	Tests your lower body balance and agility
Basic Run Plus	4.0	Wii Remote	Burns calories

Perfect 10

For this game, your Mii is surrounded by mushroom caps on which numbers appear. Your objective is to shake your hips front, back, left, or right to hit the mushrooms with the numbers that will add up to 10, as shown in Figure 6-2.

Use small, focused hip shakes, because exaggerated movements may result in you inadvertently hitting the wrong mushroom. If this ends up being the case, just hit the mushroom again to subtract it from your total, which is tracked at the top of the screen. You have 60 seconds to complete 20 rounds. For the first ten rounds, there are three mushrooms, and for the last ten, a fourth mushroom appears in front of you, compounding the arithmetic challenge. Additional challenges can be unlocked, including an Advanced level, where you have to add to 15, and an Expert level, where you have to add to 20. These levels have more rounds, but also give you a little more time to work with.

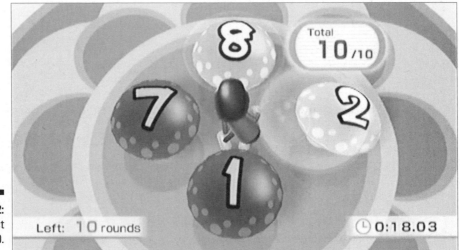

Figure 6-2:
The Perfect
10.

Having a tough time getting your children interested in practicing their arithmetic? Have them hone their skills and become math masters with this fun game, which truly puts your body and mind coordination to the test.

Scoring: Scoring is based on the time you take to complete all rounds. If you don't make it through all rounds in the time allotted, the number of rounds successfully completed will be logged for your User Ranking.

Island Cycling

For this activity, you step on the Wii Balance Board to pedal your bicycle around Wuhu Island. The Wii Remote, which you hold horizontally in front of you, serves as your virtual bike's handlebars. As a result, your bike goes in the direction that you tilt your Wii Remote. The objective is to clear all the checkpoints, which appear as flags, and return to the starting line. A small map appears in the right corner, allowing you to see the location of the flags. You can press and hold 1 on your Wii Remote to zoom out on an area of your map. The beginner course has 13 checkpoints, and additional courses can be unlocked.

Scoring: You have to clear all checkpoints for your score to be logged, which will then be recorded as the number of miles you cycled.

Rhythm Kung Fu

For this activity, you have to copy the martial arts movements of the other Mii characters in time with the rhythm. The Mii characters on the outside move first. After they complete their moves, you have to perform the same moves on the same beat. Initially, *Wii Fit Plus* instructs you on which body part to move, and you need to replicate only one move. But this activity quickly progresses through a more complex series of timed moves, and you have only your sense of rhythm to rely on. The beginner level has 35 moves. More advanced levels can be unlocked, which feature more moves. For example, the Advanced level has 42 total moves.

Scoring: Your score is determined by the number of Perfects, OKs, and Misses, worth 20, 10, and 0 points, respectively.

Driving Range

If you want to improve your golf swing and become the next Arnold Palmer or Lorena Ochoa, this game is for you. Otherwise, you may not find it to be anything special. The game assesses your center of balance and weight shift as you swing the Wii Remote, which represents a golf club. You may choose between Approach Shot, Iron, and Driver, and you have to rotate your Balance Board 90 degrees before you can begin. After you select whether you are left- or right-handed, *Wii Fit Plus* gives you a golf tutorial. After you get through that, you can start practicing. You have 20 balls to hit. As you hit them, your center of balance is traced out by a red dot during the swing, and you can also click on the Swing Analysis button at the top left of the screen to get more comprehensive feedback on how you did.

Scoring: You get ten points for each Nice Shot, five points for each OK Shot, and zero for any Missed Shot.

Segway Circuit

Always wanted to ride a Segway? Now is your chance to take a virtual version along Sugarsand Beach on Wuhu Island. As with Island Cycling, you hold the Wii Remote in front of you to control the direction of your Segway left and right. Leaning forward moves the Segway forward and leaning back makes it go in reverse. Your objective is to pop as many beach balls as possible. You can press and hold 1 on your Wii Remote to zoom out on an area of your map, which appears in the lower-right corner of your screen, to locate all the balls. Watch out for the moles, which reside in holes below the balls, as shown in Figure 6-3. Should you run into one, you will be docked five points. You can press A to have your dog pop the balls as well. A mole tries to run away with the last ball, and you have to chase him down to pop it. You have 180 seconds to complete the beginner level.

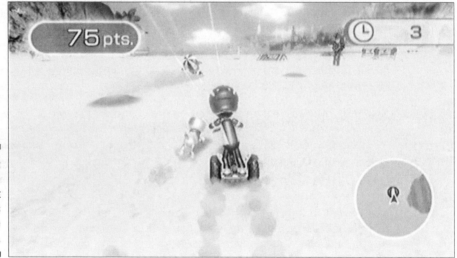

Figure 6-3:
Avoid the moles that live in holes under the beach balls.

Scoring: You receive 10 points for each beach ball popped, 100 points for catching the ball-stealing mole, and 1 point for each second remaining on your clock.

Bird's-Eye Bull's Eye

If you've always wanted to fly or you like the chicken dance, you've hit pay dirt. For this activity, you stand on the Wii Balance Board and flap your arms to reach various targets. Lean in while flapping your arms to move forward and shift your weight right or left to turn in either direction. Initially, 60 seconds are on the clock. Each target has one or more numbers on it, which represent seconds. As you land on the targets, the number you land on is the number of seconds that get added to your clock.

Scoring: After you reach the goal target, you can score 10, 20, 30, 50, or 100 (for Bull's Eye chicken) bonus points, depending on where you land. You also receive one point for each second remaining on your clock. If you don't make it to the goal target before time runs out, your distance will be logged.

Snowball Fight

Now you can engage in snowball fights without freezing your buns off. Lean left or right on the Balance Board to move out from behind your protective barrier to throw snowballs at your opponents. To hit your opponents, aim the Wii Remote at the screen and press A when the bull's-eye is on your target. Watch out for incoming snowballs. Getting hit temporarily obstructs your view, reduces your health, and results in game over if you get hit with too many. The three hearts at the bottom center of the screen represent your health. The longer you avoid getting hit by snowballs, the faster your health will refill when you do get hit. Ninety seconds are on the clock for the beginner levels. The more advanced levels, which can be unlocked, have longer durations.

Scoring: Your score is recorded as hits, and you receive one point for every target that you hit.

Obstacle Course

You step in place to walk or run, and then straighten your legs to jump over obstacles or land on mobile platforms along this obstacle course, which is reminiscent of some of the *Super Mario Bros.* worlds, especially when having to dodge Chain Chomp-like impediments, as shown in Figure 6-4. The beginner level has three platforms, with 80 seconds on the clock. When you clear a level by reaching a checkpoint, 30 seconds get added to the clock and you are lifted to the next platform. The advanced level features a more challenging course that includes icy surfaces. If you get knocked off course, you are brought back to the beginning of that platform and will have the same number of seconds on the clock as when you got thrown off. When time runs out, the game is over.

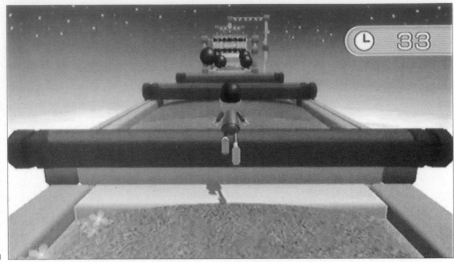

Figure 6-4:
Make Mario
jealous by
attacking
the obstacle
course
like a vid-
eogame
superstar!

Scoring: If you reach your goal, you get one point for every yard that you clear as well as one point for every second left on your clock. Otherwise, your score is recorded in yards.

Tilt City

For this activity, you have to hold the Wii Remote out in front of you and tilt it while shifting your weight on the Balance Board to tilt the three onscreen platforms to guide the dropping red, blue, and yellow balls into the matching pipe. The top platform resembles your Wii Remote and is controlled by it, whereas the two lower platforms resemble your Balance Board and are controlled by your shifting weight. The beginner level has 25 balls. More advanced levels can be unlocked, which increase the number of balls for you to coordinate. The advanced level has 40 balls.

Scoring: You receive points for each ball dropped into the correct pipe, with the balls with the Mii characters on them earning you bonus points. You also earn bonus points for dropping balls in consecutively. A perfect score is 250 on the beginner level. You do not receive or lose any points for any balls dropped into the wrong pipe.

Rhythm Parade

If you've always wanted to be in a marching band, lead the Rhythm Parade, which combines elements of a music game with stepping in place in time with the whistle. For the activity, the Wii Remote is in your right hand and the Nunchuk in your left as you stand on the Balance Board. After you start marching in time with the whistle, two circles appear onscreen, which represent your right and left hands. When the scrolling icons hit either circle, flick your hand accordingly, as you continue to step in place and lead your band through the parade. If you keep the beat, your band grows, but if you don't the band members will stop following. You know that you are keeping time if blue sparks emanate from your Mii's feet as you march, as shown in Figure 6-5. On the advanced level, the scrolling icons drop much faster.

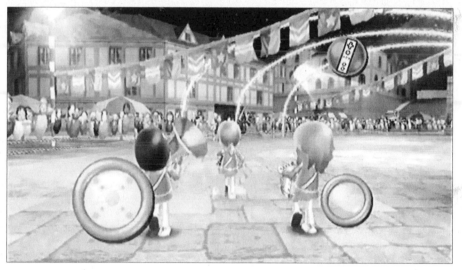

Figure 6-5: See those blue sparks or clouds? That means you are keeping time with the whistle.

Unless you have a wireless Nunchuk, when flicking your hands to get those icons as they fall into the circles, flick downward rather than upward to avoid getting hit in the face with your Nunchuk's cord.

Scoring: You receive five points for every Perfect, one point for every OK, and zero for every Miss.

Big Top Juggling

For this activity, your Mii stands on a large ball while juggling. When a ball is thrown in your Mii's direction, catch it by bringing your hand upward when the ball reaches you. Once caught, flick your hand and then your other hand to juggle it. Keep repeating these movements to keep the juggle motion going. More balls are thrown at you until you reach three balls. Watch out: Some naughty Miis are going to start throwing bombs at you. Be sure to dodge them. You have 90 seconds to accumulate points. The advanced level gives you five balls with 120 seconds on the clock.

Scoring: You receive one point for the initial successful juggle, two points for the second, three points for the third, and so on until you reach ten points, after which all successful juggles will be worth ten points, unless you lose a ball. Keep juggling those balls successfully and one of your balls will turn into an apple and be worth 20 points for every successful juggle.

Skateboard Arena

See if you can become the Tony Hawk of the Skateboard Arena. For this game, your Balance Board becomes your skateboard, and you need to turn it 90 degrees toward your television and stand sideways on it. Push off the ground with your right foot to skate forward and lean left and right to turn. If you find that you are slowing down, you can lean to the side to gain speed. The beginner level includes six levels, which progressively add more tricks for you to perform, such as riding rails and doing wheelies.

Scoring: You start with 60 seconds on the clock. You get points for skateboarding or doing tricks over the blue bars, while hitting cones deducts a point. As you complete a level, 30 seconds get added to the time you have remaining on your clock. For Level 1, you must gain 8 points to advance; Level 2, 10 points; Level 3, 10 points; Level 4, 5 points; Level 5, 7 points; and Level 6, a whopping 40 points. This equals a total of 80 points for completing the levels, and then you get 1 point for every second left on your clock.

Table Tilt Plus

This version is more challenging than Table Tilt in the Balance Games, which we describe later in this chapter. The objective is to successfully navigate your Mii-balls into the holes by tilting the floating platform by shifting your bodyweight left, right, forward, and back on the Balance Board. Movements should be subtle to prevent the balls from dropping off the table. If one or more balls drop off, you have to wait for the platform to make a 180-degree turn before your Mii-ball(s) are returned to the board, and if you had any Mii-balls left on the platform, their positions may be affected by the platform's rotation. Each table has unique contours and obstacles for you to navigate around or use to guide your Mii-balls into the goal holes, as shown in Figure 6-6. You have 60 seconds to complete all levels. This one is so challenging that we couldn't even determine how many levels are needed to complete the activity at the beginner level. Level 6 is a killer!

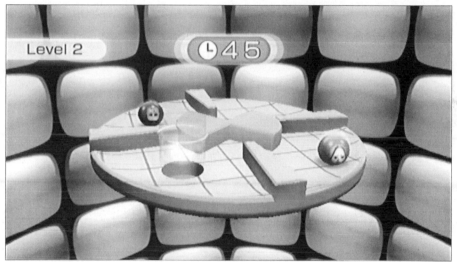

Figure 6-6:
Guide your
Mii-balls
into the goal
holes.

Scoring: You get six points for every Mii-ball successfully guided into the goal holes, which also adds six seconds to your timer. If you do manage to complete all levels, the total number of balls placed in the goal is added to the time left on the clock. Scores in the triple digits are possible but very difficult to achieve!

Balance Bubble Plus

This version of Balance Bubble is a much more challenging version than the one we describe later in this chapter. Your Mii appears in a bubble in a river, and your job is to safely navigate your Mii through the course by avoiding the river's edge and obstacles by leaning forward, backward, left, and right on the Balance Board. The farther forward you lean, the faster your Mii travels down the river, whereas leaning back will slow your Mii down. Leaning left and right steers your Mii accordingly. Keep movements subtle and control your speed until you become comfortable with the course, because you must navigate tight twists and turns, including an area where you have limited visibility and various pillars to circumvent. You have two minutes to complete the beginner course.

Scoring: This game is scored based on time, but if your Mii's bubble bursts before you reach your goal, your score is recorded in yards.

Basic Run Plus

You will put your Balance Board aside for this aerobic activity that also tests your awareness. You run the course, as you would for any of the running activities outlined in Chapter 5, but you are given a quiz about what you saw on your run at the end of the activity. You are asked questions like "Did you ever fall down?" and "How many dogs did you see?" The quiz is multiple choice.

Scoring: Your score is given as a percentage that includes your Burn Rate and Mental Focus.

Improving Your Balance with Games

Balance exercises typically focus on developing the lower body while also targeting the vestibular system. So, what is the vestibular system? Without going into too much detail, which is well beyond the scope of this *For Dummies* book or the expertise of its authors, the vestibular system comprises the structures that make up the labyrinth of the inner ear, including the cochlea, which is also part of the auditory system; the anterior, posterior, and lateral semicircular canals, which detect rotary (circular) motion; and the otolithic organs, which detect linear acceleration. These structures help control eye movements and work with the visual system to keep objects in focus when the head is in motion. They also send signals to the neural structures that control the muscles that keep you upright, allowing your body to make adjustments as needed to maintain equilibrium.

So, now you may be wondering just how you can "exercise" the vestibular system. *Wii Fit Plus* Balance Games target the vestibular system by requiring you to move your head, body, and/or eyes according to visual and auditory cues onscreen while you are being provided with feedback on your balance in real-time, allowing you to make conscious adjustments. As you continue to play these games, your vestibular system will be trained to make many of these adjustments without you consciously having to think about them, thereby improving your balance. Table 6-2 outlines *Wii Fit Plus* Balance Games.

Table 6-2	Master List of Balance Games	
Game	**MET Value**	**Equipment**
Soccer Heading	2.0	Balance Board
Ski Slalom	2.0	Balance Board
Ski Jump	2.0	Balance Board
Table Tilt	2.0	Balance Board
Tightrope Walk	2.0	Balance Board
Balance Bubble	1.5	Balance Board
Penguin Slide	2.0	Balance Board
Snowboard Slalom	2.5	Balance Board
Lotus Focus	1.0	Balance Board

Soccer Heading

The objective of this game is precisely what its title implies — to head soccer balls that other Miis kick your way. There are 80 soccer balls for the beginner level and 120 for the advanced level. Of course, there are some naughty little Miis who enjoy kicking cleats and panda heads at you, as shown in Figure 6-7, which you will have to dodge to avoid point deductions. To head the soccer balls and avoid the cleats and panda heads, you shift your weight left and right on the Balance Board, depending on which object is flying in your direction. Making contact with the soccer balls is all about getting the right timing and avoiding exaggerated movements. Your body tilts should be subtle and adjusted as soon as the ball or undesirable object is kicked your way. Unlike your Mii on the screen, you do not need to lean forward. Simply shifting your bodyweight left and right is all it takes to make contact with objects or dodge them.

Scoring: Getting hit with a cleat deducts one point from your total score, whereas those soccer-like panda heads cost you three points. Your goal should be to hit as many balls in a row as possible without getting hit with an obstacle in the process, which activates bonuses for each ball: one point for the first ball hit, two for the second, and so on until you reach a maximum of ten points per ball. The perfect score is 555 points on the beginner level and 655 on the advanced level, which is unlocked after you complete the beginner level.

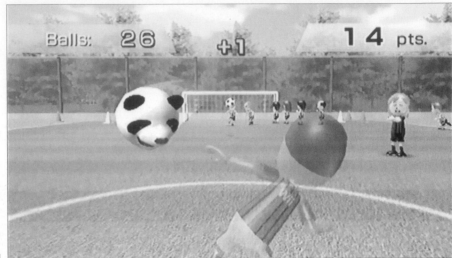

Figure 6-7:
Avoid those
panda
heads (and
cleats) or
its going to
cost points.

Ski Slalom

The objective is to guide your Mii between the red and blue flags on the course as quickly as possible without missing any. Gates that are missed result in a seven-second penalty. To guide your Mii through the slalom course, lean left and right so that your Mii skis between the flags. Movements should be subtle. Leaning too much in either direction makes it difficult to change directions quickly enough for you to guide your Mii between the flags. You can increase your speed by leaning forward and slowing down by leaning backward. To achieve an optimal speed, position yourself so that the balance point located in the upper-right corner of the screen is maintained in the blue balance bar. This may prove difficult at first. You may want to concentrate on improving your time only after you are able to comfortably guide your Mii between all the flags.

Scoring: Scoring is all about completing the course in the least amount of time possible. Every missed gate results in a seven-second penalty being added to your total time. A score of 18 seconds on the beginner setting would give you a perfect, 4-star rating. A time of 30 seconds with no missed gates would give you a perfect, 4-star rating on the advanced level, which is unlocked after repeated play of the beginner level.

Ski Jump

The objective of this game is to achieve the farthest cumulative distance (in meters) in two jumps. Like the Lotus Focus and Penguin Slide, there is no advanced setting to unlock. You start the activity with your knees bent and your body leaning forward. To achieve the optimal position, make sure the red balance dot in the upper-right corner of the screen appears in the blue balance zone (also a dot in this case); maintaining it slightly above the blue dot will allow you to gain additional speed. After your Mii reaches the red jump zone at the end of the ramp, straighten your knees as quickly as possible and stand as straight and centered as possible for the duration of the jump. The trick to mastering this is to "jump" at the right moment. If you straighten your knees too early or too late, your Mii will fall off the ramp and turn into a virtual snowball.

It may take at least a few tries to overcome your natural instincts, but remember when "jumping" you're merely extending your legs from the bent position to get your Mii airborne. If your feet leave the Balance Board at any time, *Wii Fit Plus* will end your game immediately.

Scoring: The distance you achieve on both jumps is added together for the final score. So far, the highest score we've seen online is a cumulative 404 meters; the average score appears to be between 120 and 160 meters per jump or a cumulative score between 240 and 320 meters.

Snowboard Slalom

This game requires you to reposition your Balance Board, rotating it 90 degrees clockwise, so that it better resembles a snowboard. As with the Ski Slalom, the objective is to guide your Mii between all the red and blue flags on the course as quickly as possible. Follow the arrows on the flags. The red flags have arrows that point right and the blue flags have arrows that point left, as shown in Figure 6-8. To guide your Mii accordingly, lean your body forward and backward instead of shifting your weight left and right. To achieve the optimal speed, adjust your position so that the red balance dot appears in the blue balance zone; the meter is located at the top right of the screen. All movements should be subtle, because exaggerated movement causes your Mii to stray too far off course, making it more likely that you will miss one or more turns. A miss results in a seven-second penalty being added to your time. A meter that tracks misses is located on the lower left of the screen, but you will also be alerted with a sound when you miss a turn.

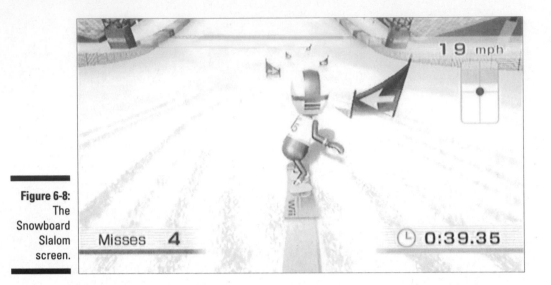

Figure 6-8:
The
Snowboard
Slalom
screen.

Scoring: Again as with the Ski Slalom, the goal is to complete the course as quickly as possible while not missing any gates. Any misses add seven seconds to your time. A time of around 18 seconds earns a 4-star rating at the beginner level and a time of about 28 seconds garners a 4-star rating at the advanced level. The advanced level is unlocked after you complete the beginner level.

Table Tilt

This game is perhaps one of the most challenging of the Balance Games, though not nearly as challenging as Table Tilt Plus discussed earlier in this chapter. Table Tilt can be thought of as the opposite of the classic wooden labyrinth puzzle, where instead of trying to keep a ball out of the holes, the goal is to get one or more balls in a hole. To successfully complete this activity, you must complete eight different levels before time runs out.

To tilt the floating platform and guide your Mii-balls into the holes, you shift your bodyweight left, right, forward, and back on the Balance Board. Holding your arms out to the sides may help improve your balance. Movements should be subtle to prevent the balls from dropping off the table. Although many platforms have a curved edge, which acts as somewhat of a protective buffer, it doesn't take much to tilt the platform enough for those Mii-ball(s) to drop. Don't worry: This won't end the game, but it will cost you some precious time, because you will have to wait for the platform to make a 180-degree turn before your Mii-ball(s) are returned to the board. Furthermore, if you had any Mii-balls left on the platform, their positions may be affected by the platform's rotation, potentially setting you further back. However, sometimes dropping balls can be advantageous, because it can facilitate getting others in the holes. Each table has unique contours, and with practice, you learn how to avoid or use them to your advantage. After you complete Level 8, your Mii-balls cheer you on as they return to their Wii form, as though a curse has been lifted.

Scoring: Completing a level scores you 10 points and adds an additional 20 seconds to the clock. There are a total of eight levels to complete, and one point is awarded for each second you have left at the end. A score of 0 to 29 nets you one star; 30 to 79, two stars; 80 to 99, three stars; and 100+, four stars.

Tightrope Walk

Ever want to walk a tightrope? Now you can do so without worrying about going splat. For this activity, you walk in place to guide your Mii across a high wire straddled between two skyscrapers while other Miis cheer you on from the target building. Your Mii will move relative to your center of balance, so when your center of balance is off, your Mii will lean too far to one side and will start sweating and becoming distressed. You will have to set them right before advancing; otherwise they will plummet to Wii oblivion (at least until you try again). You will also have to watch out for that iron jaw advancing toward you who is hungry for some Mii, as shown in Figure 6-9. Help your Mii jump over those jaws by straightening your legs at just the right time. It is best to jump when those iron jaws are directly in front of your Mii. Things become more challenging on the advanced and expert settings. On the advanced setting, your Mii has three iron jaws to jump over and floating bird feathers at the start make it difficult to see your Mii on the screen. On the expert setting, you will not only have those iron jaws to contend with, but also wind gusts that can push you off the rope if you don't compensate for them. The advanced setting becomes available after you complete beginner mode and the expert setting becomes available after the advanced setting has been completed.

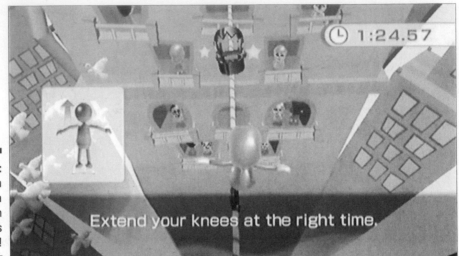

Extend your knees at the right time.

Scoring: You have two minutes to cross the high wire. The faster you cross it, the higher your rating. If you don't cross it in the allotted time, you automatically fall off the rope and your score will be recorded in yards instead of time.

Balance Bubble

In this game, your Mii appears in a bubble in a river. Your job is to safely navigate your Mii through the course by avoiding the river's edges and staying away from the bees, which are all too happy to burst your Mii's bubble, causing your Mii to plunge into the water, ending the game. If you let your Mii get too close to the river banks without correcting course, it becomes distressed and starts trembling before the bubble finally pops.

You guide your Mii down the river by leaning forward, backward, left, and right on the Balance Board. The farther forward you lean, the faster your Mii travels down the river, whereas leaning back slows down your Mii. Leaning left and right steers your Mii accordingly. It is best to keep movements more subtle and control your speed until you become comfortable with the course, as there are some twists and turns to navigate. One way you can avoid the bees is to pass them quickly, which is easier to do on the beginner level than the advanced one. This game also has an advanced setting, which is unlocked after you complete beginner mode. On the advanced level, there are more bees, and they seem to be more aggressive — sort of like Africanized bees versus honeybees on the beginner level.

When you reach the fork in the river, it is best to veer right, as that path is considerably wider than the one on the left. Of course, if you'd like more of a challenge, go left to take the narrower and less forgiving course.

Scoring: This game is scored based on time, much like the Tightrope Walk, and you are allotted 90 seconds to complete the board. If you run out of time or your Mii hits the river's edge or gets stung by a bee, your Mii's bubble will burst, your score will be recorded in yards, and you will receive a one-star rating. If you successfully make it to the mouth of the river, your score will be recorded in time.

Penguin Slide

In this fast-paced game, your famished Mii is standing on an iceberg and donning a penguin suit. Luckily, the fish are flying! They are literally jumping out of the water, just tempting you to eat them. You catch them by quickly tilting the iceberg left and right. Like the Ski Jump and Lotus Focus, there is no advanced setting to unlock, but this game is challenging enough even without one.

You need to shift your body weight left and right to tilt the iceberg in the direction necessary to catch the fish. As you tilt the iceberg, your Mii begins to slide downward in the direction of the tilt. If you aren't careful with how far you tilt, your Mii will slide off the iceberg completely and you'll have to wait several seconds before your Mii can hop back on again. Staying in the center of the iceberg as much as possible prevents your Mii from sliding into the icy water and allows you to access fish on both sides of the iceberg more easily, ensuring you optimize your fish-catching potential. But keep in mind that not all fish are created equal! Be sure to pay close attention to the large red fish, as shown in Figure 6-10, because they are quite the catch. Once one of these red fish appears beneath the iceberg, take note of which side of the iceberg it eventually dives out of sight on, as it will surface shortly thereafter above the iceberg on the same side. Catching these red fish is considerably more challenging because the iceberg doesn't tilt high enough for you to catch them. You will have to hoist yourself toward them, which you do by positioning your Mii below one of these fish on the iceberg and then quickly tilting the iceberg in the opposite direction. It takes some practice to be able to perform this maneuver consistently, but the extra points are well worth the effort.

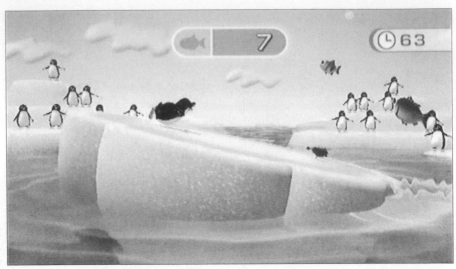

Figure 6-10:
The Penguin
Slide
screen.

Scoring: The blue fish are worth one point, the green fish are worth two points, and the challenging red fish are worth +points.

Lotus Focus

This game is perhaps the most deceptively simple of all *Wii Fit Plus* activities. Lotus Focus, or Zazen, is a key Zen Buddhist practice, and is essentially the act of sitting as still as possible. What differentiates this seated meditation movement from the more popular "couch potato" — besides the absence of salty snacks — is its focus on concentration. In its *Wii Fit Plus* form, Lotus Focus challenges you to maintain unwavering focus on an onscreen candle — the slightest twitch causes air to rush over your candle, possibly extinguishing it! If your candle's flame is snuffed out, so is your game.

Unlike the other balance games, you begin Lotus Focus by sitting on the Balance Board with your legs folded and the palms of your hands resting on your knees. Be sure your back is straight and you breathe smoothly. Once the test begins, you must remain as focused and motionless as possible while breathing normally. To make things more difficult, a virtual moth will fly about and various sound effects will play at different times to try to distract you.

Zazen is typically performed with a variety of leg configurations, so feel free to experiment with different seated positions.

Scoring: Scoring is all about remaining focused and well balanced for as long as possible, up to 180 seconds, at which point you are declared a champion.

Part II

EA Sports Active: Personal Trainer

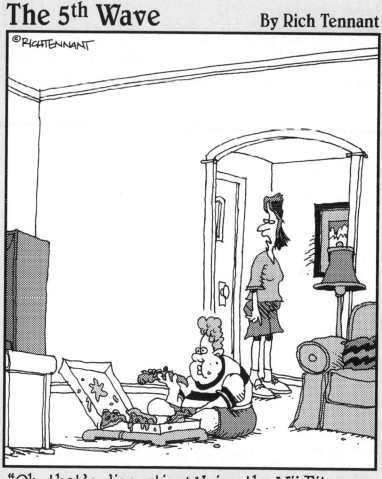

The 5th Wave — By Rich Tennant

©RICHTENNANT

"Oh, that's disgusting! Using the Wii Fit as a tray table for your pizza!"

In this part . . .

*E*A Sports Active: Personal Trainer is the one fitness game that comes closest to challenging Wii Fit's dominance as the top videogame fitness title, and, in this part you find out why. You get to know what's in the *EA Sports Active: Personal Trainer* package, including the Leg Strap and Resistance Band, as well as how to navigate around the software and create your first fitness profile. Next, you are introduced to the upper body, lower body, cardiovascular, and sports exercises, and learn how to perform them properly. Finally, you learn how to work with the preset exercise routines, as well as how to create personalized routines that are optimized for your specific needs and goals.

Chapter 7

Getting Started

The original *Wii Fit* redefined the fitness videogame genre with its unique peripheral, the Balance Board, which uses your center of balance to track movements. Turn to Chapter 1 for more on the Balance Board and its unique capabilities. Although it was widely popular and well-received, *Wii Fit* has shortcomings that later exercise-based games sought to correct. Most notably, *Wii Fit* lacks the capability to continuously stream exercises or select a workout routine, which can leave you feeling lost and as though you are spending more time navigating menus than actually working out. Although this has been addressed with *Wii Fit Plus,* it doesn't provide nearly as robust a portal for setting and customizing workouts as the vastly popular *EA Sports Active: Personal Trainer,* which lives up to the promise of giving you a 20-minute workout. Working out with *EA Sports Active: Personal Trainer* is much like working out with a quality exercise DVD, with the added bonuses of having your movements tracked and providing real-time guidance and encouragement. As its title suggests, you truly feel as though you have a personal trainer at your side. *EA Sports Active: Personal Trainer* also generates new routines based on your goals every time you work out, keeping workouts interesting and fresh.

This chapter provides you with all the information you need to get started using your *EA Sports Active: Personal Trainer.* You find out how to assemble, use, and care for the tools that come with the program — the Resistance Band and Leg Strap. You also discover how to use the software, including navigating the menus and calendars, create your Fitness Profile, incorporate the Balance Board, and take the 30 Day Challenge.

Exploring What's in the Box

When you purchase your *EA Sports Active: Personal Trainer,* you receive the software, which features more than 25 different exercises and sports-based activities (see Chapter 8 for the complete list); a ribbon-style Resistance Band, which you have to assemble (as outlined in the next section); and a Leg Strap that comes with an Adjustment Strip, allowing you to adjust the size of the strap, if necessary. Figure 7-1 shows the contents of the *EA Sports Active: Personal Trainer* bundle. Try not to feel overwhelmed by the accessories in the bundle. They each serve a specific purpose. The Leg Strap remains on your leg for all *EA Sports Active: Personal Trainer* activities, and its sole purpose is to house the Wii Nunchuk for exercises that require tracking your lower body movements, such as Dancing, Kick-ups/High Knees, and Squats. The Resistance Band is used to increase the intensity of many upper body exercises, such as upright rows, bicep curls, and both shoulder raises and presses. The Resistance Band has a resistance level of .20 mm, which is considered very low. If you want to increase your resistance level, you can purchase stronger bands. See Chapter 13 for more on Resistance Bands, including some options.

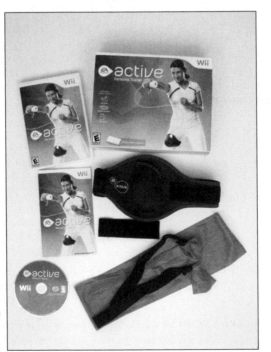

Figure 7-1:
The contents of
*EA Sports
Active:
Personal
Trainer.*

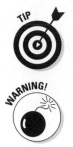

To extend the life of your Resistance Band, which is constructed of very thin latex, we recommend storing it in a cool, dry place, such as a sealable bag or plastic box with lid, and putting a little baby powder or cornstarch on it between uses to prevent moisture buildup.

Allergy alert! The Resistance Band is constructed of a natural latex rubber and has a powder coating to which small latex particles can attach, so if you have a latex allergy, do *not* open the package. Latex-free alternatives are available. Because latex allergies can appear at any time and may worsen with repeated exposure, use of the Resistance Band should be discontinued immediately if any sensitivity is noticed, as life-threatening reactions, albeit extremely rare, are possible. According to the EA Active Web site, the Leg Strap is composed of neoprene, a synthetic rubber, and has a natural rubber backing, but no latex; however, latex is a natural rubber and caution may still be warranted. Neoprene itself can lead to an allergic reaction in some individuals; therefore, if you have a neoprene, latex, or other rubber allergy, you should find an alternative. This may prove a bit challenging, but some people have reported success using stretchy sports sweat headbands, for instance, to keep the Wii Nunchuk in place.

Gearing Up

The Resistance Band package contains one red Resistance Band and two black straps. Putting these three components together to form one cohesive unit is a snap — well, maybe more of a fold and a pull — that takes less than a minute. Follow these steps:

1. **Spread the red Resistance Band out on a smooth, flat surface, such as a table or the floor, and take one of the black straps and place it under the flattened red band, roughly two to three inches from one end of the band.**

   The big loop of the black strap should be facing you, as shown in Figure 7-2.

2. **Fold the big loop over the red Resistance Band, as shown in Figure 7-3.**

3. **Pull the big loop of the black strap through the smaller loop, as shown in Figure 7-4, and keep pulling until the resulting knot is tight and secure.**

4. **Repeat these steps with the other black strap, and you will be good to go.**

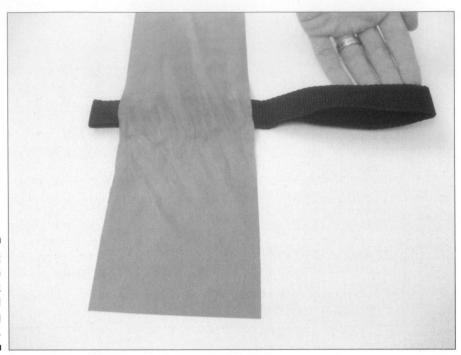

Figure 7-2:
The big loop of the black strap should be facing you.

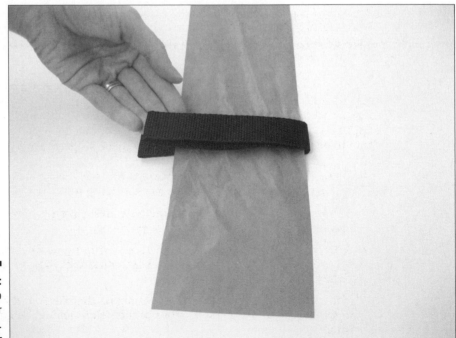

Figure 7-3:
The big loop folded over the band.

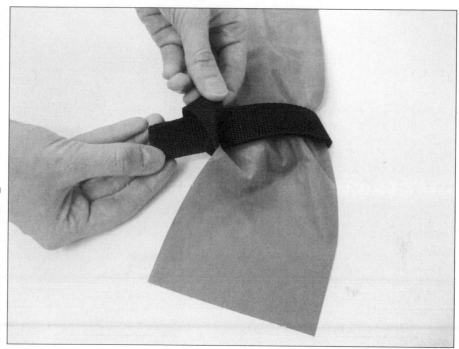

Figure 7-4:
The big loop gets pulled through the smaller loop, creating a knot when pulled tight.

The Leg Strap is 28 inches wide and comes with a 5-inch adjustment strip. The *EA Sports Active: Personal Trainer Instruction Booklet* refers to this strip as a hook and loop fastener, but you are probably more familiar with its trade name of Velcro, which we refer to it as throughout the book. The adjustment strip can be used to either shorten or extend the strap, the latter of which is not discussed in the *Instruction Booklet*. The Leg Strap works best if you wear form-fitting pants or shorts. Loose pants, such as jogging pants, or slick fabrics don't allow the Leg Strap to be tightened enough, making it prone to slippage during your workout, which can get quite annoying. Try on the Leg Strap to ensure you get a proper fit. Follow these steps:

1. **Place the Leg Strap around your right leg, with the pouch facing forward and the opening of the pouch facing up.**

   The Leg Strap should be high enough so that it stays put, but not low enough to interfere with bending your knees.

2. **After you've found the proper position, bring the ends together and thread the long strap through the black plastic buckle, as shown in Figure 7-5.**

   You can thread it through either opening on the plastic buckle, but the hook (rough) and loop (soft) sides of the Velcro should be facing each other.

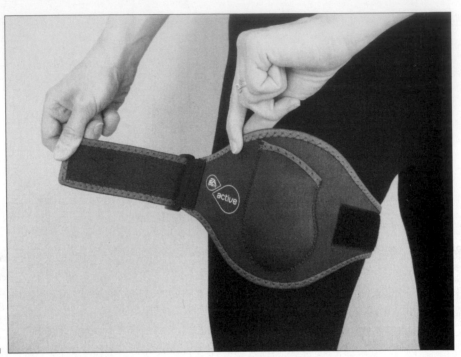

Figure 7-5:
Proper
position
of the Leg
Strap.

3. **Pull the long strap until it is snug, but not so tight that you cut off your circulation, and secure the Leg Strap by pressing the hook and loop sides of the Velcro together.**

   The Leg Strap should be comfortable upon squatting, and if positioned correctly, the pouch will be sitting on top of your thigh when your legs are at a 90-degree angle during the squat. If not, loosen the strap and readjust until you find the proper position and fit.

Is the Leg Strap too small? You can add up to an additional three inches to it by using the Velcro adjustment strip. Follow these steps:

1. **Spread the Leg Strap out on a flat surface with the pouch facing you.**

2. **Expand the overall length by attaching the loop side of the Velcro adjustment strip to the hook side of the Velcro on the Leg Strap.**

   Placement of the adjustment strip determines how much length you gain.

3. **After placing the Leg Strap in the correct position on your leg, so that the pouch is facing forward and the opening of the pouch is facing up, thread the Velcro adjustment strip through the black plastic buckle.**

Is the Leg Strap too large? Whip out that Velcro adjustment strip and follow these four steps to shorten it:

1. **Spread the Leg Strap out on a flat surface with the pouch facing you.**

2. **Shorten the overall length by folding a segment of the strap over itself, as shown in Figure 7-6.**

   The amount that is folded is the amount by which the strap is shortened.

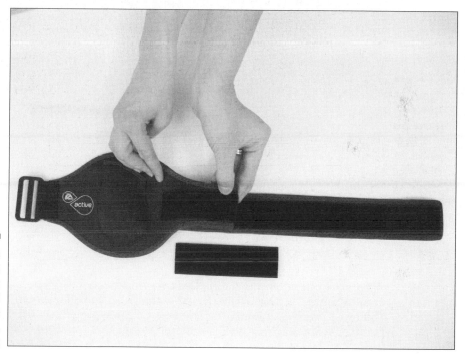

Figure 7-6:
The Leg Strap being shortened through folding.

3. **Take the Velcro strip and press the hook side firmly down onto the loop sides of the Leg Strap so that the strip straddles the folded and unfolded segments of the Leg Strap, as shown in Figure 7-7.**

4. **Try the shortened Leg Strap on for size, and if necessary, adjust the fold and secure the Velcro strip.**

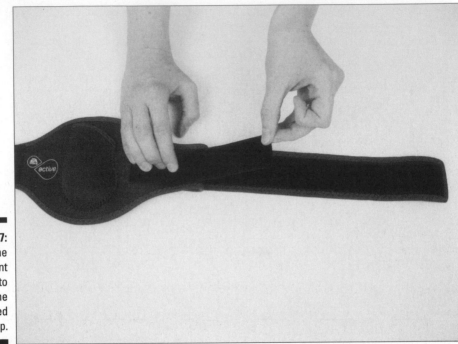

Figure 7-7:
Use of the
adjustment
strip to
secure the
shortened
Leg Strap.

Creating Your Fitness Profile

Although you can proceed directly into your workout by selecting the green Guest Pass in the lower-right corner of the Fitness Profile screen, shown in Figure 7-8, we recommend that you take a minute to create a fitness profile. Establishing a fitness profile is required to track your progress in a fitness journal and to participate in the 30 Day Challenge. Setting up a profile takes just a few minutes, and you can edit or delete your fitness profile any time. You can create up to five fitness profiles, allowing your family or friends to get in on the action.

Establishing your Fitness Profile

To create your fitness profile, hover over a Create New card on the main menu and press A. Doing this brings you to the Personal Stats screen. Enter your gender, age, height, and weight by hovering over the appropriate arrows and pressing A or by holding down the A button while hovering over the slider in the middle of the scale and moving your Wii Remote left or right until the proper value appears in the slider. The minimum and maximum values for the stats are:

- ✔ 5 to 95 years for age
- ✔ 3 to 8 feet for height
- ✔ 30 to 300 pounds for weight

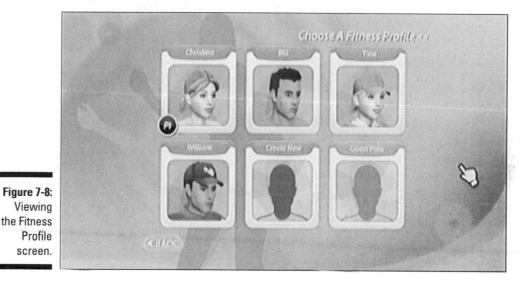

Figure 7-8:
Viewing
the Fitness
Profile
screen.

Because this information is used to calculate your projected calorie burn for each activity, it is in your best interest to be as accurate as possible. Don't be discouraged if you weigh more than 300 pounds. Although discovering this arbitrary weight limitation in the software may be disappointing, it won't impede you from performing the exercises, and getting in a good workout is ultimately all that matters. You can even incorporate the Wii Balance Board if you weigh up to 330 pounds, which is the weight limit of the Board; however, the Balance Board is optional and not using it does not limit the activities available to you. When you are satisfied with your personal stats, hover over Next and press A. Doing this pulls up an avatar for you to customize.

Customizing your avatar

A male or female avatar appears on the screen, depending on which gender was selected on the Personal Stat screen. None of the other information entered on that screen will affect your avatar's looks, unlike *Wii Fit Plus,* which weighs you and shapes your Mii to its best guess. Eight simple steps are required to customize your avatar. After you make your selection for each category, press Next to go to the next screen. If you decide at any point during the customization process that you want to change one or more of your selections, just click the Back button at the bottom of the screen until you get to the screen(s) that you want. Follow these steps to customize your avatar:

1. **Select your avatar's body type.**

   You can use the arrows or pull the bar in the middle of the scale to the left (for thinner) or to the right (for heavier) to make your selection; even the heaviest option does not make for a very heavy looking avatar.

2. **Select your avatar's skin color from the six available options.**

3. **Select a hair style.**

   There are 6 choices for male avatars and 11 for female avatars. You can access additional options for female avatars by pressing A while hovering over the arrow on the right. If you prefer an option on the first screen, click the arrow on the left to get back to it.

4. **Select one of the six available hair colors.**

5. **Dress your avatar.**

   There are 18 options for men and 20 for women. Click the arrow on the right to scroll through the myriad options and the one on the left to access previously displayed options.

6. **Select a hat.**

   Eleven are available to choose from. Of course you also have the option of resisting temptation and going hatless.

7. **Choose to go with or without sunglasses.**

   Five fashionable sunglass options are available.

8. **Select your avatar's sneakers.**

   Five options are available. No barefoot avatars allowed, so no shoes, no service!

Now you can create your Fitness Journal. After your final selection has been made, an onscreen keyboard appears. Use the keyboard to enter your name. Unless your name is conveniently "Name," make sure you hover over the Backspace button and press A until you've deleted all the letters from the top window. If you want uppercase letters, hover over Shift and press A. Now hover over the letters you need and press A; you can enter a total of ten characters. After your name has been entered, select OK. Congratulations! You now have your very own Fitness Journal!

Editing your Fitness Profile

You can edit or delete a fitness profile any time. Just go to the main menu and select Fitness Profile. Then click on the profile you wish to edit. Doing this opens the screen containing your fitness profile. This screen has four options. The last two options are Edit Fitness Profile and Delete Fitness Profile. If you select the latter, you are asked to confirm this decision. Should you select Yes, the profile is history. If you choose to edit your profile instead, you go through the same menu that you went through to establish the profile, including the Personal Stats screen and each of the eight avatar customization screens. After you finish making your modifications, which concludes with the shoe selection, your changes are automatically saved and you are transported back to your fitness profile — no clicking of heels needed.

Earning trophies

You can earn a total of 30 trophies in *EA Sports Active: Personal Trainer.* The trophies are outlined in Table 7-1. Trophies are awarded to celebrate your achievements and milestones, and can be accessed through your fitness profile by selecting View My Trophies.

Table 7-1	Trophies
Name	*Achievement*
Go-Getter	Completed Workout 1 of the 30 Day Challenge
Half Way There	Completed Workout 10 of the 30 Day Challenge
Fitness Superstar	Completed Workout 20 of the 30 Day Challenge
30 Day Champion	Completed the 30 Day Challenge in 30 days or less
Dear Diary	Completed 1st Journal entry receiving all 3 check marks
Trend Setter	Completed 7th Journal entry receiving all 3 check marks
Checking In	Completed 30th Journal entry receiving all 3 check marks
Getting Fresh Air	Earned an activity level rating of over 400 in the other Activity survey
Fitness 101	Completed 101 Exercises

(continued)

Table 7-1 *(continued)*

Name	Achievement
Tennis Pro	Completed 200 swings in Tennis
Born to Skate	Completed 100 jumps in In-line Skating
Running in the Mix	Ran 25 laps on the track
Slugger	Swung the bat 200 times in Baseball
Volleyball Champ	Completed 200 hits in Volleyball
Fists of Fitness	Punched 500 targets in Boxing
Dance Fever	Completed 1,000 steps in Dancing
Slam Dunk	Completed 200 baskets in Basketball
Squat Master	Completed 100 squats
GOAAAAAL!	Completed 1 goal
Goal Achiever	Completed one Calorie Goal, one Workout Hours Goal, and one Workouts Goal
Workout Buddies	Worked out with a friend
Completionist	Completed every exercise at least once
Feel the Burn	Burned 100 Calories
Fitness Inferno	Burned 1,000 Calories
Fuel for The Fire	Burned 10,000 Calories
50 Strong	Completed 50 Workouts
Going for Gold	Earned a Gold Medal
Making it Mine	Created and completed a Custom Workout
Power Hour	Worked out for a total time of 1 Hour
Ten out of Ten	Worked out for a total time of 10 Hours

Navigating the Main Menu

EA Sports Active: Personal Trainer features numerous options that are accessible from the main menu (see Figure 7-9) after choosing your fitness profile. The menu options are: Journal, Fitness Profile, 30 Day Challenge, Preset & Custom Workouts, Help & Settings, and Info, each of which is selectable by hovering over the option with your Wii Remote and pressing the A button. If you log in under a Guest Pass, the Journal and 30 Day Challenge options become selectable, but you are asked to create or load a Profile to be able to continue with your selection. Each of the possible menu options is summarized in Table 7-2, and described in further detail elsewhere in this chapter.

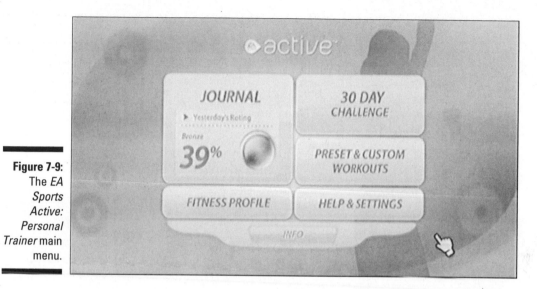

Figure 7-9:
The *EA Sports Active: Personal Trainer* main menu.

You can press the Home button on your Wii Remote at any time to bring up the Home menu. The Home menu options enable you to return to the Wii system menu, reset the console, check Wii Remote battery levels, or change your Wii Remote settings. For more information on these options, refer to your *Wii Operations Manual.*

Table 7-2	Main Menu	
Menu Option	*Description*	*Available to Guest Pass?*
Journal	Track your fitness progress	No
Fitness Profile	Select your active profile for the current session	Yes
30 Day Challenge	Creates a workout and rest schedule for a single 30-day period	No
Preset & Custom Workouts	Tackle single preset or custom workouts with or without a friend	Yes
Help & Settings	Modify settings, watch videos, check the Balance Board, and see the game's Credits	Yes
Info	Ten bite-sized tips and key information	Yes

Keeping Your Fitness Journal

The Fitness Journal is used to track your workout progress. The Fitness Journal main page, shown in Figure 7-10, shows your daily checklist, medals achieved for the day, and trainer feedback. You can also access your goals, profile, and calendar. In the following sections, we examine each of these Journal components more closely.

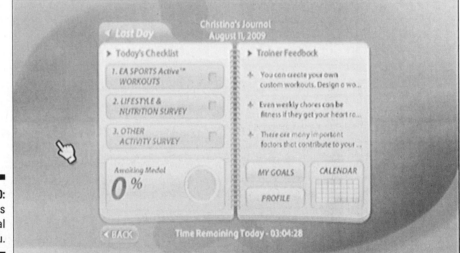

Figure 7-10: The Fitness Journal main menu.

The Checklist

The Checklist includes three items: EA Sports Active Workouts, the Lifestyle & Nutrition Survey, and the Other Activity Survey. To have all three checked off in your Fitness Journal for the day, you need to complete a workout and both surveys. Selecting EA Sports Active Workouts allows you to choose a workout to complete. You can select one from your 30 Day Challenge or a preset or custom workout. The custom workout option is only available to you after you've created your own routine. We discuss how to do this in Chapter 9. After you complete your workout, EA Sports Active Workouts are checked off for the day.

The Lifestyle & Nutrition Survey asks you ten questions about how well you are taking care of yourself outside of *EA Sports Active: Personal Trainer* and gives you trainer tips. For example, you are asked how many sugar-containing drinks you consumed the day before, how stressed you are currently feeling, and how many hours of quality, uninterrupted sleep you received. To answer these and other questions, click on the + or – signs on the left-hand page to make your selection and press Next when you are satisfied with your answer.

When you complete the survey, your answers are displayed on the left and trainer tips based on your responses appear on the right, as shown in Figure 7-11. You also see a Graph option on the bottom of the left-hand page of your Fitness Journal. If you select it, you see a monthly graph that plots out your answers to the lifestyle factors that you were queried on as well as what your goals should be based on the trainer tips provided. There are a total of ten graphs, one for each question, so you have to click the arrows on the bottom of the graph to scroll through to see them all. You can also opt to see a weekly graph by clicking the Weekly Graph button in the lower-right corner of the graph. If you click that button again, it reverts back to the monthly graph. To exit the graph screen, select the Close X tab in the upper-right corner. Doing this brings you back to your survey results. If you are finished with this page, click Done. Your results are saved and the Lifestyle & Nutrition Survey is checked off.

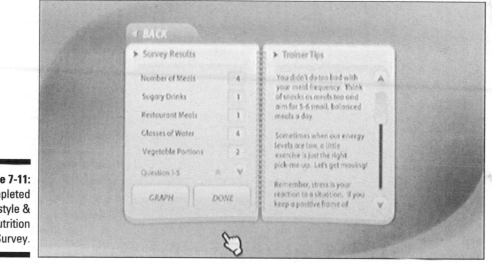

Figure 7-11:
A completed
Lifestyle &
Nutrition
Survey.

Through the Other Activity Survey, *EA Sports Active: Personal Trainer* rewards you for physical activities performed outside of the program, whether they are sports-based or regular daily activities, such as yard work. After you select the Other Activity Survey from your Fitness Journal's main menu, you come to a screen where there are three physical activity tips and instructions on the left and Graph and Add Activities options on the right. If you select Add Activities, you come to a screen where you can choose from 15 activities, which you have to scroll through by clicking the up and down arrows or dragging the slider up and down, as shown in Figure 7-12. After you find an activity you want to add, click on it. This brings you to a screen that asks you how much time you spent doing the activity and to rate your intensity level. Activity time is added in five-minute increments. Make your selections by pressing the + and – signs. The right-hand page for each selected activity contains a definition of the activity and/or an explanation of its general intensity level. You can add numerous activities to the survey, and you will see Total Time and the Average Intensity for all activities you have added to the activity selection menu. After you've added all your activities, click Submit. This step brings you back to your Fitness Journal's main menu. As with the Lifestyle & Nutrition Survey, if you select Graph, you can see your activities plotted out and can select between a Weekly and Monthly Graph.

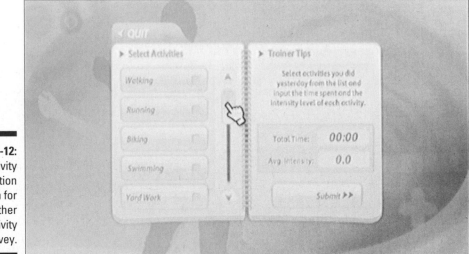

Figure 7-12:
Activity
selection
screen for
the Other
Activity
Survey.

Daily medals

Each day that you use your Fitness Journal, you are awarded a gold, silver, or bronze medal, depending on your performance during the workout, your responses to the daily Lifestyle & Nutrition survey, and your reported activity levels outside of *EA Sports Active: Personal Trainer*. At the bottom of the Fitness Journal screen, notice the countdown timer. Fortunately, after this time lapses, your *EA Sports Active: Personal Trainer* will not self-destruct, but you will have run out of time to complete your workout. This means you will receive no medal or whatever medal was obtained by completing one or both of the surveys. Generally, doing the workout first is best. The surveys can be completed later without penalty, allowing you to get a gold medal even after time runs out. Also, although you won't receive a medal on days that none of the items on your checklist is completed, you can still receive a gold medal on designated rest days as long as you complete the surveys.

If you click on your daily medal, you can get an overview of your Journal Stats, including your current age, height, weight, calories burned, average activity level, total workout time for the day, average daily rating for medals (bronze, silver, or gold), and average health rating.

Goals, Profile, and Calendars

EA Sports Active: Personal Trainer allows you to set the following three goals:

- ✔ **Calories** sets how many calories you'd like to burn over a certain period of time (500 calories in seven days, for example).

- ✔ **Hours** sets how many hours you'd like to work out over a designated period of time (such as ten hours over 17 days).

- ✔ **Workout** sets how many workouts you'd like to complete over a certain period of time (five workouts over seven days, for example).

You can select goals for all three, some, or none. As long as your Fitness Profile is active, these goals can be tracked in any area, and *EA Sports Active: Personal Trainer* can give you feedback on whether you are achieving your goals. If you find that your goals were too easy or overly ambitious, you can reset or delete them at any time. Just click on My Goals in the lower left of the right-hand page of your Fitness Journal, select the goal you want to reset or delete, and then follow the prompt to make your selection.

When you select Profile from the Fitness Journal menu, you have three options: View My Trophies; Edit Fitness Profile; and Delete Fitness Profile. Each of these options is discussed in detail earlier in this chapter.

Your Fitness Journal Calendar pulls up a monthly calendar that shows your workout history, medal history, and rest days. For detailed information on a particular day, click on the day you want to see. Doing this pulls up your Fitness Journal entry for that day. You can scroll through the days before and after it by clicking on the Last Day or Next Day tabs at the top of the screen.

Working Out

Now that you've created your Fitness Profile and familiarized yourself with the main menu and Fitness Journal, it's time to start working out. You can choose between the 30 Day Challenge, or single session Preset & Custom Workouts with or without a friend.

As shown in Figure 7-13, there are three basic elements to a single player workout screen. In the upper left is calories burned so far. To the upper right is the current length of the workout. In the middle is trainer feedback. Finally, depending upon the exercise, you may also see an exercise guide/indicator to the left of your avatar and the trainer to the right showing you what to do next.

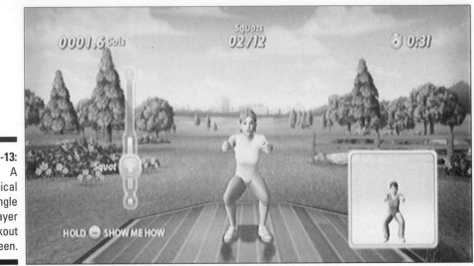

Figure 7-13:
A typical single player workout screen.

Figure 7-14 shows the basic screen elements when working out with a friend. At the top of each half of the screen is the individual calories burned. In the top center of the split screen is both players' common goal. In the bottom center of the split screen is the current length of the workout. Finally, depending upon the exercise, you may also see each of your trainers toward the bottom of your respective halves of the screen showing you each what to do next.

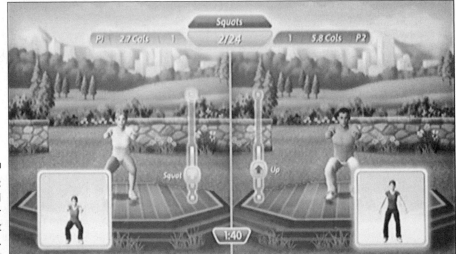

Figure 7-14:
A typical two player workout screen.

After you start an exercise, the Wii Remote's + button brings up the Pause menu options, holding the 1 button opens and closes the Jukebox, and holding the – button opens and closes Show Me How.

30 Day Challenge

The 30 Day Challenge is a great way to help you set a goal and structure a realistic timeline to achieve it. As you improve with each workout, *EA Sports Active: Personal Trainer* adapts to keep both the challenge and your motivation level high. New workouts are prepared each day, made up of various exercises that are tailored to the intensity level of your choosing. Of course, as is the hallmark of any good workout program, body parts worked are rotated, and rest days are strategically placed throughout your 30 Day Challenge's calendar, as shown in the Weekly Calendar View in Figure 7-15.

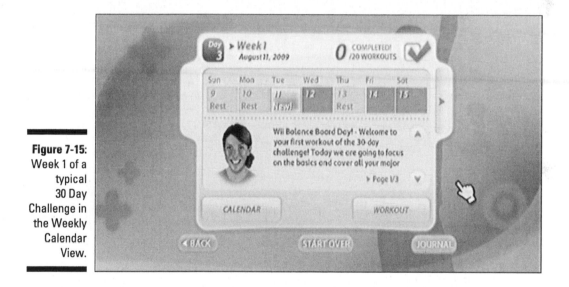

Figure 7-15: Week 1 of a typical 30 Day Challenge in the Weekly Calendar View.

The Weekly Calendar View is the main screen for your 30 Day Challenge. You can see what days you have to work out, what days you should rest, and whether you missed a day. Your trainer provides a summary for each day's activities. You can select Workout to begin that day's activities, or go back and play a previous day's activities. Selecting Calendar gives you a longer view of your workout history and schedule up to your Finish Day, which is 30 days from your start date, though you can keep playing the increasingly misnamed 30 Day Challenge up until day 90, at which point the Challenge must be restarted.

The first day you begin a new workout during the 30 Day Challenge, you will be prompted to choose one of three intensity levels (low, medium, or high), whether you wish to use the Wii Balance Board, and what type of music you want to listen to.

The choice of intensity level appears only the first time you start your first workout in a 30 Day Challenge, so we recommend that you set your first 30 Day Challenge to Low intensity, which still provides for some tough workouts. After you finish your first 30 Day Challenge, you can consider moving up to the Medium intensity level if you feel you are ready for it.

Upon successfully completing a 30 Day Challenge, you can go to EA's official Web site, `http://www.easportsactive.com/blog.action?month=7&year=2,009`, and get a 30 Day Challenge badge that you can proudly display on your favorite social-networking or other Web site. While there, you can also check out other fun activities related to the 30 Day Challenge and *EA Sports Active: Personal Trainer* in general.

Preset & Custom Workouts

Don't feel like tackling a complete 30 Day Challenge or want to do something completely different on a particular day, like playing only your favorite exercises and activities? Selecting Preset & Custom Workouts from the main menu allows you to create, save, and access your own Custom Workouts, or choose from a selection of preset workouts designed around a particular goal. See Chapter 8 for a thorough description of each of the exercises, and Chapter 9 for more on creating your own Custom Workouts and routines.

Using Help & Settings

Have a regret about something you set in the 30 Day Challenge and want to change it? Want to see video of one of the exercises in action? You can do all this and more from the Info menu, which appears after selecting Help & Settings from the main menu. The options are: Settings, Tutorial Videos, Wii Balance Board Check, Credits, and Back.

Selecting Tutorial Videos brings up a selection of every *EA Sports Active: Personal Trainer* exercise activity as demonstrated by either the selected male or female trainer, and its corresponding summary information. Credits shows a list of the many talented individuals who made *EA Sports Active: Personal Trainer* possible. Back returns you to the main menu. Settings and Wii Balance Board Check are described in the next sections.

Settings

Selecting Settings from Help & Settings reveals four options: Workout Settings, Audio Settings, Create My Playlist, and Back, the latter of which returns you to the preceding menu option. Selecting Workout Settings allows you to turn Wii Balance Board support on or off, your Personal Trainer to Male or Female, and the game's Measurement Units to Metric or Imperial. Audio Settings allows you to change Music Volume, sound effects volume, and your Playlist options: All Songs, Modern Beats, Guitars & Alternative, Custom, Electronica, Dance Club, and Hip Hop & Urban. Audio Settings also features a second tab for Trainer Settings, which changes their Speech Volume and how much, if any, feedback they provide. Create My Playlist allows you to customize what music you hear from the 41 available tracks.

Wii Balance Board

Selecting Wii Balance Board Check allows you to verify the normal operating status of your Balance Board. If your Balance Board has not already been synced to your Wii, you must do that before proceeding. Follow the onscreen instructions or refer to Chapter 1 for more information on setting up the Balance Board with your console.

Use of the Balance Board is optional and provides alternative ways to perform certain exercises and activities. Unfortunately, due to the technical limitations of the board, it is not available in the multiplayer portion of the game.

Getting Fit with a Friend

Although the original *Wii Fit* kicked off the Wii fitness phenomenon, it certainly wasn't perfect, with one of its biggest omissions being a lack of multiplayer support beyond its running games. Among the many ways *EA Sports Active: Personal Trainer* distinguishes itself from the competition is by allowing you to perform all its exercises with a friend. To select this mode, go to the Preset & Custom Workout screen via the main menu and select Workout with a Friend. After you adjust the settings to your liking and begin, a split-screen view displays your avatar and friend's working out side-by-side, with your respective trainers showing what to do next. This mode is a great way to find that little bit of extra motivation to power through that day's workout as you and your friend compete not only for individual goals, but to contribute to your team goal.

You will need a second Wii Remote and Nunchuk, as well as an EA Sports Active: Accessory Pack, or equivalent, to be able to perform all the exercises and activities. So grab the pack and a friend and get to it!

Chapter 8

Performing the Exercises

· ·

· ·

*W*ith more than 25 exercises, *EA Sports Active: Personal Trainer* provides a multitude of workout options. If you become bored with following a regular workout routine, then you can give the program's sports drills a try, which include fun activities such as dancing, volleyball, and baseball. Regardless of which activities you choose, you are guaranteed to break a sweat while still having fun, and you may just forget that you are working out.

This chapter provides an overview of all the exercises that are available in *EA Sports Active: Personal Trainer*. We've broken them out by upper body, lower body, cardio, and sports drills, allowing you to easily find exercises to target specific body parts and goals. Although this chapter provides guidance on how to perform each activity, *EA Sports Active: Personal Trainer* lets you watch a video demonstration of each exercise before undertaking it, ensuring that you never feel lost. In this chapter, you discover all that *EA Sports Active: Personal Trainer* has to offer.

Working Your Upper Body

The upper body exercises focus on your back, shoulders, arms, chest, and abdominals. For these exercises, you use the Resistance Band, which provides a bit of tension, forcing your muscles to work just a little bit harder. Exercising your upper body increases strength, improves posture, ensures mobility of the joints, and builds bone density — all of which become especially important as you age. Plus, the work you put into sculpting your upper body won't go unnoticed, because these gains are often the most visible.

To ensure the optimal and safe performance of several exercises, you have to become familiar with the Standing Hip Hinge position. To achieve this position, stand on one foot and bring your other knee upward. Place your fingers in your hip crease. After you bring your knee down, stand with your feet shoulder-width apart and place your hands on your hips with your thumbs forward. Squeeze your elbows together to open your chest. Hold this position and bend forward, pushing your tailbone away from your chin. Keep your shins vertical and look straight ahead. As with all the exercises in this chapter, you can refer to the *EA Sports Active: Personal Trainer* tutorial video under the Help & Settings menu on the Standing Hip Hinge to see this technique in action.

Alternating Bicep Curls

This exercise primarily works the bicep muscle of each arm. To get your biceps pumped, follow these steps:

1. **Stand with your feet shoulder-width apart and knees slightly bent, with the Resistance Band under the arches of both feet and a handle in each hand.**

   The Wii Remote should be in your right hand and the Nunchuk in your left.

2. **Place your hands at your sides and hold the handles with your palms facing forward.**

3. **Curl your right hand up in a semicircular motion until your forearm touches your biceps, keeping your elbows immobile and close to your sides at all times.**

   As shown in Figure 8-1, actively contract your biceps at the top of the movement, making sure not to bend your wrist.

4. **Lower your hand to the starting position and then curl up with your left hand.**

   Repeat the sequence for the indicated number of repetitions.

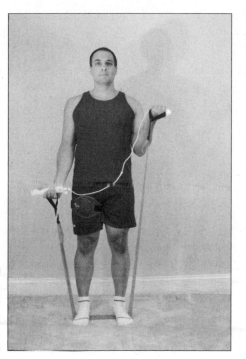

Figure 8-1:
Apex of
Alternating
Bicep Curls.

Alternating Cross Knee Punches

Although this exercise focuses on the upper half of your body, the complete motion brings together both halves at its apex, targeting your abdominals. Follow these steps:

1. **Hold the Wii Remote in your right hand and the Nunchuk in your left and stand with your feet shoulder-width apart and your knees slightly bent.**

2. **Extend your arms out in front of your body, keeping them at shoulder height and parallel to the floor.**

3. **Lift one knee up and across your body to hip height while simultaneously bringing your arms down toward that knee, as shown in Figure 8-2.**

4. **Tighten your abdominal muscles as your arms meet your knee.**

    Repeat, alternating sides for the indicated number of repetitions.

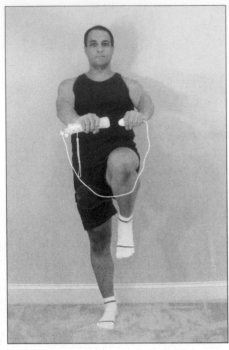

Figure 8-2:
Apex of
Alternating
Cross Knee
Punches.

Alternating Shoulder Presses

This exercise primarily works your deltoids, which are the muscles that give your shoulders their rounded contour. Follow these steps to start building shoulders that look great sans shoulder pads:

1. **Place the Resistance Band under the arches of both feet and grasp the handles.**

   The Wii Remote should be in your right hand and the Nunchuk in the left. Make sure your feet are shoulder-width apart and your knees slightly bent.

2. **Hold your hands at ear level, elbows down, wrists in line with the elbows, and palms facing forward.**

   Keep your chest open and your eyes focused straight ahead.

3. **Straighten one arm and press your hand overhead until your arm reaches full extension.**

   Pause when the Wii Remote or the Nunchuck is pointed at the ceiling, as shown in Figure 8-3.

   Remember to keep your core tight as you press.

4. **When you bring your hand back to the start position, actively pull your arm downward.**

   Repeat, alternating sides for the indicated number of repetitions.

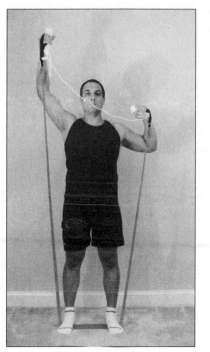

Figure 8-3:
Apex of
Alternating
Shoulder
Presses.

Alternating Triceps Kickbacks

Kickbacks work the triceps muscle at the back of your arm. Exercising these muscles helps eliminate arm jiggle. Follow these steps for toned triceps:

1. **Stand with your feet shoulder-width apart and knees slightly bent, with the Resistance Band under the arches of both feet and a handle in each hand.**

   The Wii Remote should be in your right hand and the Nunchuk in the left.

2. **As described in the beginning of this chapter, do a Standing Hip Hinge and hold your torso at a 45-degree angle.**

3. **Keep your abdominals tight and back flat throughout the movement.**

4. **Lift your elbows to your ribcage and pin your elbows to your side, keeping them there until all of your repetitions are finished.**

5. **With your palms facing each other, straighten one arm out behind you so that it is parallel to your body.**

6. **Point the Wii Remote or Nunchuk at the floor at the top of the motion, as shown in Figure 8-4.**

7. **Bend your arm back to the starting position and repeat, alternating sides for the indicated number of repetitions.**

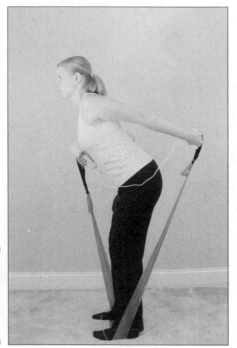

Figure 8-4: Apex of Alternating Triceps Kickbacks.

Bent Over Rows

This exercise primarily works the *rhomboids,* or muscles of the upper back. Make people envious of your back by following these steps:

1. **Stand with your feet shoulder width apart and knees slightly bent, with the Resistance Band under the arches of both feet and a handle in each hand.**

   The Wii Remote should be in your right hand and the Nunchuk in the left, both pointing toward the floor.

2. **As described in the beginning this chapter, do a Standing Hip Hinge and hold your torso at a 45-degree angle, or, for a greater challenge, parallel to the floor.**

   Keep your abdominals tight and back flat throughout the movement.

3. **Focus on your back muscles as you slowly pull your hands to your lower rib cage, leading with your elbows and keeping your arms close to your sides as you pull up.**

   The Wii Remote and Nunchuk should become parallel to the floor, pointing forward. Keep your gaze straight ahead. Your head and neck should be slightly relaxed. Keep your shoulders down and shoulder blades retracted to fully engage your back muscles, as shown in Figure 8-5.

4. **When you reach your chest, pause, and then slowly lower your arms back to the start, again pointing the Wii Remote and Nunchuk toward the floor.**

   Repeat for the indicated number of repetitions.

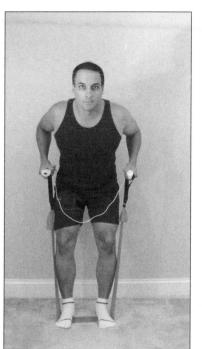

Figure 8-5:
Apex of
Bent Over
Rows
performed
at a
45-degree
angle.

Bent Over Rows with Triceps Kickbacks

This exercise combines bent over rows with triceps kickbacks to target both your upper back and the back of your upper arms. Follow these steps to perform this exercise:

1. **Stand with your feet shoulder-width apart and knees slightly bent, with the Resistance Band under the arches of both feet and a handle in each hand.**

2. **Hold the Wii Remote in your right hand and the Nunchuk in the left, with both facing each other and pointing toward the floor as you straighten your arms.**

3. **As described in the beginning of this chapter, do a Standing Hip Hinge and hold your torso at a 45-degree angle, or, for a greater challenge, parallel to the floor.**

   Keep your abdominals tight and back flat throughout the movement.

4. **Focus on your back muscles as you slowly pull your hands to your lower rib cage, leading with your elbows and keeping your arms close to your sides as you pull up.**

5. **Keep your head and neck slightly relaxed and your eyes looking forward. Keep your shoulders down and shoulder blades retracted to fully engage your back muscles.**

6. **When you reach your chest, hold your elbows to your rib cage and pin your elbows to your side.**

7. **With your palms facing each other, straighten one arm out behind you parallel to your body.**

   The Wii Remote or Nunchuk should be pointed at the floor at the top of the motion.

8. **Bend your arm back to the starting position and repeat for the other arm.**

   Repeat this sequence beginning with the bent over row for the required number of repetitions.

Bicep Curl with Shoulder Press

This exercise targets both your biceps and deltoids. Follow these steps to perform the exercise:

1. **Stand with your feet shoulder-width apart and knees slightly bent, with the Resistance Band under the arches of both feet and a handle in each hand.**

The Wii Remote should be in your right hand and the Nunchuk in your left.

2. **Place your hands at your sides and hold the handles with your palms facing forward.**

3. **Curl your hands up in a semicircular motion until your forearms touch your biceps, keeping your elbows fixed at your sides at all times.**

   Actively contract your biceps at the top of the movement, making sure not to bend your wrists.

4. **After a brief pause, move your hands to ear level, keeping your elbows down, wrists in line with the elbows, and palms facing forward.**

   Your chest should be kept open and your eyes focused straight ahead.

5. **Straighten both arms and press your hands overhead until your arms reach full extension.**

6. **Pause after the Wii Remote and Nunchuk are pointed at the ceiling.**

   Remember to keep your core tight as you press.

7. **Actively pull your arms downward as you lower and turn your hands back to the finish position for the bicep curl.**

8. **Lower your arms back to the beginning of the bicep curl and repeat the entire sequence for the required number of repetitions.**

Bicep Curls with Upright Rows

This combination exercise targets your biceps, trapezius (muscles at the side of the base of the neck), and deltoids. Get to curling and rowing by following these steps:

1. **Stand with your feet shoulder-width apart and knees slightly bent, with the Resistance Band under the arches of both feet and a handle in each hand.**

   The Wii Remote should be in your right hand and the Nunchuk in your left.

2. **Place your hands at your sides and hold the handles with your palms facing forward.**

3. **Curl your hands up in a semicircular motion until your forearms touch your biceps, keeping your elbows pinned to your sides at all times.**

4. **Actively contract your biceps at the top of the movement, making sure not to bend your wrists.**

5. **After a pause, lower your hands back down to the front of your thighs as you open your chest and pull your shoulders down and back.**

6. Face your palms over your thighs and relax your arms in front of you.

7. Lift your hands up toward your chin, leading the movement with your elbows, which should finish above your shoulders.

8. Pause at this top position and then slowly lower your hands back to your thighs. Repeat the entire sequence starting at the bicep curl for the required number of repetitions.

Front Shoulder Raises

This exercise focuses on the front part of the muscle at the top of the shoulder, the deltoid. Take one step closer to developing well-defined shoulders by following these steps:

1. Stand with your feet shoulder-width apart and knees slightly bent, with the Resistance Band under the arches of both feet and a handle in each hand.

   The Wii Remote should be in your right hand and the Nunchuk in your left.

2. Hold your arms in front of your thighs and face your palms toward each other.

3. With your elbows slightly bent and your shoulders down and back, lift your arms straight out in front to shoulder height, making sure you keep your thumbs pointed up.

4. Lower your arms back to the starting position and repeat for the required number of repetitions.

Lateral Shoulder Raises

This exercise focuses on the lateral part of the muscle at the top of the shoulder, the deltoid. Try these steps for shapely shoulders:

1. Stand with your feet shoulder-width apart and knees slightly bent, with the Resistance Band under the arches of both feet and hold each handle.

   The Wii Remote should be in your right hand and the Nunchuk in your left.

2. Bend your elbows to 90 degrees (parallel to the floor) and face your palms toward each other.

3. Lift your arms up, maintaining the 90-degree bend, making sure to lead with your elbows.

Keep your shoulders down and back as you raise your arms to shoulder height, as shown in Figure 8-6.

4. **Slowly lower your arms back to the starting position and repeat for the required number of repetitions.**

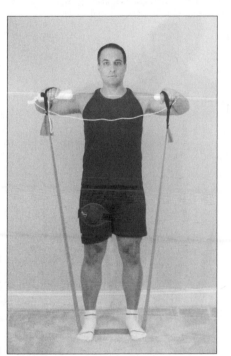

Figure 8-6:
Apex of
Lateral
Shoulder
Raises.

Upright Rows

Upright Rows work the trapezius, deltoids, and, to a lesser degree, biceps. Follow these steps to tone your upper body:

1. **Stand with your feet shoulder-width apart and knees slightly bent, with the Resistance Band under the arches of both feet and a handle in each arm.**

   The Wii Remote should be in your right hand and the Nunchuk in your left.

2. **Place your hands at your sides, open your chest, and pull your shoulders down and back.**

3. **Face your palms over your thighs and relax your arms in front of you.**

4. **Lift your hands up toward your chin, leading the movement with your elbows, which should finish above your shoulders, as shown in Figure 8-7.**

5. Pause at this top position, then slowly lower your hands back to the front of your thighs.

6. Repeat for the required number of repetitions.

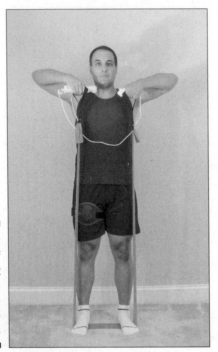

Figure 8-7:
Apex of
Upright
Rows. Note
the posi-
tion of the
elbows.

Working Your Lower Body

The lower body exercises focus on your gluteal and leg muscles. For these exercises, you place the Nunchuk in the pocket on the Leg Strap, which allows your leg movements to be tracked. Although the work you put into your lower body may not be as readily apparent to others, this area should not be neglected; otherwise, your body may end up looking out of proportion. Working your lower body also helps improve balance, which can go a long way in preventing any injuries from unstable footing.

Alternating High Knee Reverse Lunges

This exercise not only places stress on the quadriceps, hamstrings, and glutes, but also requires a great deal of balance and coordination. Follow these steps:

1. **Stand with your feet close together, slightly less than shoulder-width apart.**

   The Wii Remote should be in your right hand and the Nunchuk in the Leg Strap around your upper-right thigh.

2. **Place your hands on your hips, or, as your balance improves, alternate pumping your arms with each lunge.**

3. **Take a large step backward onto the ball of your right foot in a reverse lunge.**

   Lower until your left front thigh is nearly parallel to the floor. Keep your torso upright and steady by keeping your abdominals tight.

4. **Push off both your front and back foot, and straighten your front leg.**

5. **Bring your back leg through to the front of your body, lifting your knee to hip height, as shown in Figure 8-8.**

   Contract your glutes to stabilize yourself.

6. **Find your balance and repeat for the other side.**

   Continue alternating sides for the required number of repetitions.

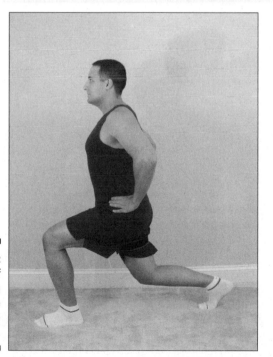

Figure 8-8:
Apex of
Alternating
High Knee
Reverse
Lunges.

Alternating Lunges

This exercise challenges your balance and coordination, while placing stress on your quadriceps, hamstrings, glutes, and adductors, or the muscles of your inner thigh. Build a rock-solid bottom by following these steps:

1. **Stand with your feet close together, slightly less than shoulder-width apart.**

2. **The Wii Remote should be in your right hand and the Nunchuk in the Leg Strap around your upper-right thigh.**

3. **Place your hands on your hips, or, as your balance improves, alternate pumping your arms with each lunge.**

4. **Take a large step forward with your right leg and lunge toward the floor.**

   Keep your torso upright and steady. Allow the trailing left knee to bend. Do not allow your front knee to move beyond your toes.

5. **When both legs make 90-degree angles, as shown in Figure 8-9, push off your front foot and return to the start.**

6. **Find your balance and repeat for the other side. Continue alternating sides for the required number of repetitions.**

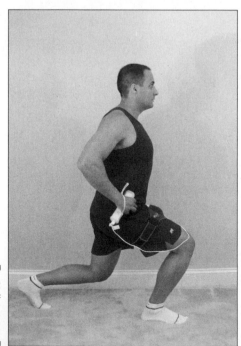

Figure 8-9:
Apex of
Alternating
Lunges.

Alternating Side Lunges

This exercise places most of its stress on the outer thigh and hip area, as well as the glutes. Follow these steps to perform the exercise:

1. **Stand with your feet and knees close together, slightly less than shoulder-width apart.**

   The Wii Remote should be in your right hand and the Nunchuk in the Leg Strap around your upper-right thigh.

2. **Place your hands on your hips or out in front to help with your balance.**

3. **Take a large step to the right side and lunge toward the floor.**

4. **Descend until your right thigh is almost parallel to the floor, but make sure your knee does not pass your toes.**

5. **Sit back into your glutes, keeping your back straight, your hips square, and your bodyweight on your heels.**

   Keep your trailing left foot securely on the floor, as shown in Figure 8-10.

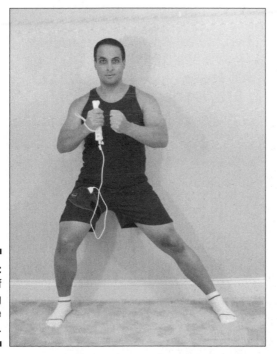

Figure 8-10:
Apex of
Alternating
Side
Lunges.

6. **Push off and return to the start.**

7. **Repeat for the other side, continuing to alternate sides for the required number of repetitions.**

Alternating Side Lunges with Toe Touches

This combination exercise places most of its stress on the outer thigh, hip area, and the glutes. It also challenges your flexibility and coordination. Work your legs by following these steps:

1. **Stand with your feet and knees close together, slightly less than shoulder-width apart, and place the Wii Remote in your right hand and the Nunchuk in the Leg Strap around your upper-right thigh.**

   Make sure that the Wii Remote is pointing toward the ceiling.

2. **Take a large step to the side and lunge toward the floor. Descend until your leading thigh is almost parallel to the floor.**

   Make sure that your knee does not pass your toes.

3. **Sit back into your glutes, keeping your back straight, your hips square, and your bodyweight on your heels.**

   Keep your trailing foot securely on the floor. Pause. (See Figure 8-11.)

4. **Tilt the Wii Remote to point directly at the floor.**

5. **Return to an upright torso position, push off through your foot, and return to the start.**

   Repeat for the other side, continuing to alternate sides for the required number of repetitions.

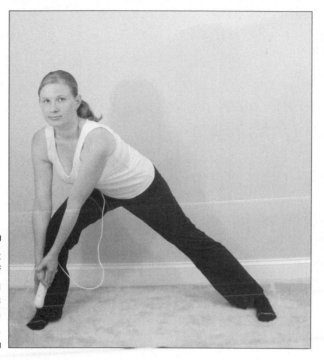

Figure 8-11:
Apex of
Alternating
Side Lunges
with Toe
Touches.

Alternating Standing Knee Crunches

This exercise challenges your balance and muscle control abilities. Become well-balanced by following these steps:

1. **Stand with your feet and knees close together, slightly less than shoulder-width apart.**

   The Wii Remote should be in your right hand and the Nunchuk in the Leg Strap around your upper-right thigh.

2. **Place your hands firmly in front of your stomach.**

3. **Lift your right knee to the front of your body at hip height, while bending over at the waist, as shown in Figure 8-12.**

4. **Place your foot back down and repeat for the required number of repetitions, alternating knees.**

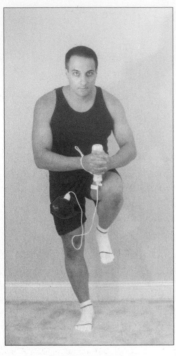

Figure 8-12:
Apex of
Alternating
Standing
Knee
Crunches.

Jump Lunges

Jump Lunges are a *plyometric,* or explosive type of exercise that works your entire upper leg and glutes. Follow these steps:

1. **Place the Wii Remote in your right hand and the Nunchuk in the Leg Strap around your upper-right thigh.**

2. **Stand tall in a lunge position, with one leg forward and one back.**

3. **Bend both knees and lower yourself down to preload your muscles.**

4. **Jump up as high as you can, pushing the floor away and driving your arms to generate more power.**

5. **At the apex of the jump, reverse the direction of your legs, back to front, and front to back.**

    Switching the legs occurs in mid-air before landing. Land as softly as possible, keeping your body under control.

6. **Line up your knees before beginning your next jump.**

7. **Repeat as indicated.**

   Watch the placement of your front knee and both feet when landing, keeping them pointed forward at all times.

Jump Squats

This exercise is another plyometric exercise that works the upper thigh, glutes, and calves but also places a great deal of stress on your entire cardiorespiratory system. Follow these steps to perform the exercise:

1. **Place the Wii Remote in your right hand and the Nunchuk in the Leg Strap around your upper-right thigh.**

2. **Stand with your feet wider than shoulder-width apart and place your hands at your sides.**

3. **Keep your back straight and head up as you squat down.**

4. **When your thighs are almost parallel to the floor, push the floor away from you as you jump upward as high as you can.**

5. **Fully straighten your legs in the air, and then land on the balls of your feet.**

   You should challenge your muscles and cushion your landing by landing as softly as possible and bending your knees as you sit back into your glutes. Also, try to land evenly with both feet; they should make contact with the floor at the same time.

6. **Immediately reverse the motion and perform another jump.**

   Repeat as indicated. As you fatigue, you can generate more power by leading with your arms.

Side To Side Jumps

This plyometric exercise works your entire lower body and cardiovascular system. Get your heart pumping by following these steps:

1. **Place the Wii Remote in your right hand and the Nunchuk in the Leg Strap around your upper-right thigh.**

2. **Enter a quarter squat position with your feet parallel and shoulder width apart.**

Bring your arms back slightly prior to jumping.

3. **With your feet and knees close together, jump to the side, extending all your joints in the air.**

   Drive your arms upward to generate more power and assist you in achieving maximum distance and height.

4. **Land softly into the squat position, toe to heel, as you sit back into your glutes.**

   Try to land evenly with both feet, so that they make contact with the floor at the same time.

5. **Pause briefly and perform another jump.**

   Repeat as indicated.

Squat & Hold

This exercise works your upper thigh and glutes, but especially challenges your muscular endurance. Test your endurance by following these steps:

1. **Place the Wii Remote in your right hand and the Nunchuk in the Leg Strap around your upper-right thigh.**

2. **Stand with your feet shoulder-width apart and your toes and knees slightly pointing outward.**

3. **Place your hands out in front of you for balance, keeping your back straight and head up.**

4. **Squat down until your thighs are almost parallel to the floor.**

5. **With your knees tracking over your toes, back straight, and chest open, hold this position for the time indicated.**

Squats

Often referred to as the king of exercises, squats involve your quadriceps, hamstrings, and glutes, but also stress your entire cardiorespiratory system. Master the squat by following these steps:

1. **Place the Wii Remote in your right hand and the Nunchuk in the Leg Strap around your upper-right thigh.**

2. **Stand with your feet shoulder-width apart and your toes and knees slightly pointing outward.**

3. **Put your hands on your hips or out in front of you for balance.**

4. **Keep your heels in contact with the floor and your knees lined up over your toes as you squat down until your thighs are almost parallel to the floor.**

   Be sure to keep your back straight and head up as you squat down.

5. **Squeeze your glutes as you power yourself back up, and repeat for the required number of repetitions.**

 Never push off on your knees with your hands to help yourself back up when performing any type of squat exercise. Doing so may compromise your posture and potentially injure your back or knees.

Squats with Calf Raises

Squats with Calf Raises provide the powerful benefits of regular squats with additional focus on your calves, challenging your balancing abilities. Follow these steps:

1. **Place the Wii Remote in your right hand and the Nunchuk in the Leg Strap around your upper-right thigh.**

2. **Stand with your feet shoulder-width apart and your toes and knees slightly pointing outward.**

3. **Put your hands on your hips or out in front of you for balance and keep your knees lined up over your toes as you squat down until your thighs are almost parallel to the floor.**

   Keep your back straight and your head up as you squat.

4. **As you reach the bottom position of the squat, pause, and lift your heels off the floor in a calf raise, as shown in Figure 8-13.**

5. **Lower your heels and stand back up, pushing the floor away from you as you return to the starting position.**

   Repeat the sequence for the required number of repetitions.

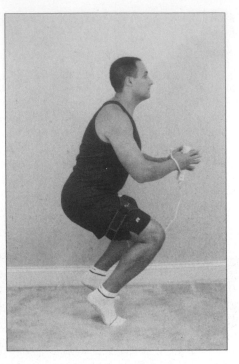

Figure 8-13:
Bottom
position of
Squats with
Calf Raises.

Standing Twists

Standing Twists are among the least challenging exercises, which make them good for warming up, helping to space out difficult exercises, or simply for increasing flexibility. Despite its relative simplicity, as with all exercises, care must be taken to perform this movement in a controlled and deliberate manner to minimize the risk of injury. Get to twisting by following these steps:

1. **Stand with your feet shoulder-width apart and knees slightly bent, with the Wii Remote in your right hand and the Nunchuk in your left.**

2. **Extend your arms in front of your body at shoulder height, keeping them parallel to the floor.**

3. **Twist your torso, carefully accelerating through the movement while keeping your arms steady.**

4. **Pause briefly before accelerating in the opposite direction.**

   Be sure to turn your torso as a unit, never allowing your arms to get ahead of you. Repeat for the required number of repetitions.

Increasing Your Heart Rate with Cardio

Cardiovascular exercises are important to preserve heart and lung function. These activities can help burn body fat, lower blood pressure, and improve your cholesterol profile by increasing high-density lipoprotein (HDL) cholesterol levels. It is thought that HDL transports cholesterol to the liver, where it is passed from the body rather than dangerously building up in the blood vessels. Although the breathlessness and repetitive motions of cardio for extended periods of time may be off-putting to some, *EA Sports Active: Personal Trainer* makes cardio fun by engaging your mind. The activities are easy to follow and enable you to take them at your own pace, helping to ensure you stick with your fitness program.

Cardio Boxing

EA Sports Active: Personal Trainer offers two Cardio Boxing activities: Heavy Bag and Punching Targets. These activities work your cardiovascular system while conditioning your upper body, especially your arms and shoulders, and require you to punch targets using a variety of combinations, including straight punches, crossover punches, and heavy bag punches. As you become more experienced, the combinations become more complex. Be sure to keep your legs shoulder-width apart and your knees slightly bent for these activities. You hold the Wii Remote in your right hand and Nunchuk in the left. A typical boxing screen is shown in Figure 8-14.

While you needn't move your feet during these activities, you can burn more calories and get a better cardiovascular workout if you mimic the foot movement of actual boxers. To do this, stay on the balls of your feet and bob up, down, left, and right when throwing punches.

Heavy Bag

This activity focuses on developing speed and force, and you will have to dole punches quickly to reach the target. Be sure to fully extend your arms with each punch to get the most out of this exercise. After you hit the target the required number of times, the heavy bag becomes unhinged if you've delivered enough punishment, so don't hesitate to blow off some steam when engaging in this activity.

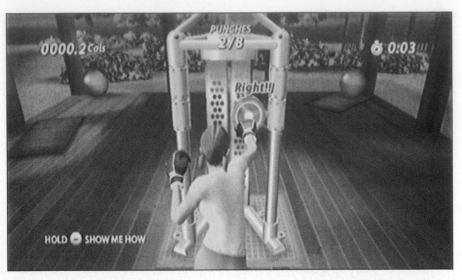

Figure 8-14:
A typical
boxing
screen
featuring
Punching
Targets.

Punching Targets

As its name implies, this activity requires you to punch targets as they appear, and you use straight punches and crossover punches. For the straight punches, hit the red targets straight on with the correct hand so that your arm is extended directly in front of you at roughly shoulder height. To perform crossover punches, hit the blue targets by punching across your body with the opposite hand. Left targets will be hit with your right hand and right targets with your left hand. Your arm should extend across your body at roughly shoulder height. To put force behind both straight and crossover punches, snap at your elbow at the end of the swing. If you deliver enough force with your punches, the targets will break. Demolishing the targets is fun and an indication that you are working at a higher intensity level, ensuring you are maximizing the benefits of this activity.

Wii Balance Board

When you use the Balance Board to do Cardio Boxing, the activity also involves your legs, making the activity more like Kick Boxing. When the activity starts, you should be standing on the board with your feet shoulder-width apart and knees slightly bent. The activity combines kicks and knee strikes with punches on the heavy bag. When kicking the heavy bag, kick out with your right or left foot. Be sure to pull your leg up high with each kick to maximize the workout, and return your foot fully to the board after each kick. To do knee strikes, raise your right or left leg knee high to strike the bag. Pull your knee up high with each kick to maximize the benefit.

Cardio Dancing

These activities could be described as a *DanceDanceRevolution* for the arms, as you will have to perform several arm movements in time to the beat of the music by following the directional arrows as they fall into the green zone on the screen, as shown in Figure 8-15. The Cardio Dancing activities are short, consisting of 56 moves total, regardless of which level is undertaken. In the middle of these dance sequences, you encounter a specialty move, such as Do the Shopping Cart, Start that Lawnmower, or Wave the Lasso. You won't be following directional arrows for these sequences, just mimicking the movements of your onscreen classmates, and the movements will be straightforward. While you aren't required to move your feet for Cardio Dancing, you will find these activities much easier to perform if you bounce with the beat of the music. For stability, be sure to keep your feet shoulder-width apart and your knees slightly bent.

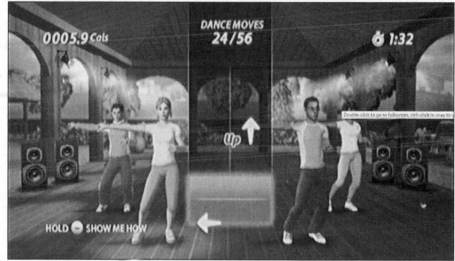

Figure 8-15:
Follow the movement for each directional arrow, as indicated onscreen, when it falls into the green zone.

Wii Balance Board

When you use the Balance Board to do Cardio Dancing, the activity also involves your legs, and you will be stepping on and off the board while also moving your arms. When the activity starts, you should be standing on the board with your feet shoulder-width apart and knees slightly bent. Watch the onscreen indicators, which help you keep up with the cardio dance moves. Try to keep beat with the music and the background dancers.

Track

Running around a track dates back to the ancient Greeks and was the only event at the Olympics in 776 BCE, which is the first Olympics for which we have a written record. Since then, track and field activities, also commonly referred to as athletics, have evolved considerably. *EA Sports Active: Personal Trainer* has numerous track-based activities, including High Knees, Kick Ups, running, and walking. You can use the walking activity to warm up or cool down, and if you are looking for a more intense activity, give running, High Knees, or Kick Ups a try. A typical track screen is shown in Figure 8-16.

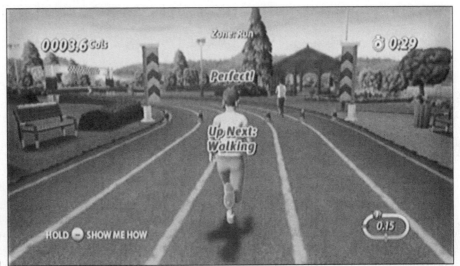

Figure 8-16: A typical track screen.

High Knees

When you do High Knees, bring your knees up high enough when you raise each leg so that your thigh is parallel with the ground. Be sure to maintain your posture by keeping your back straight and shoulders back. It will look like you are marching in place. If you want to be a true fitness soldier, be sure to pump your arms.

Kick Ups

When you do Kick Ups, keep your steps light and stay on the balls of your feet. Each time you raise a leg, drive your heel back toward your glutes. If you are doing this correctly, your leg may lightly kick the back of your thighs. For maximum benefit, pump those arms, which burns more calories and helps improve your balance and posture.

Running

When running, be sure to lean forward slightly. Doing this places your center of mass on the front part of your foot, facilitating your foot's spring mechanism. Be sure to pump your arms as well. Upper body motions compensate for the motions of the lower body and are important for keeping the body in rotational balance. The more force you exert with your lower body, the more exaggerated your arm pumping should be to keep this balance.

Walking

When you are told to walk, gently walk in place. You will see the characters walk onscreen, so you will know that you are doing the right movement. Be sure to swing those arms!

Having Fun with Sports

Sports are a great way to work out. The sports-based drills in *EA Sports Active: Personal Trainer* target both upper and lower body muscle groups, and many of the activities give you a solid cardiovascular workout. Even if you've never played sports, don't hesitate to give these drills a try. Who knows, they may just inspire you to try your hand at the real thing.

Baseball

On the virtual baseball diamond, you perform several reflex-oriented activities, including swinging a bat, and catching and throwing a ball, all designed to challenge your upper body. Most of the movements are performed with the Wii Remote in your right hand and the Nunchuk in your left, though you can incorporate more lower body work and increase the challenge through the use of the Balance Board. An example of a typical Baseball screen is shown in Figure 8-17.

Batting

To bat, hold the Wii Remote in your hand and swing when you see the ball being pitched toward you. Hitting the ball with enough power gives you a home run, while hitting the ball lightly with give you an infield hit. For greater effect, twist your body into the ball as you swing.

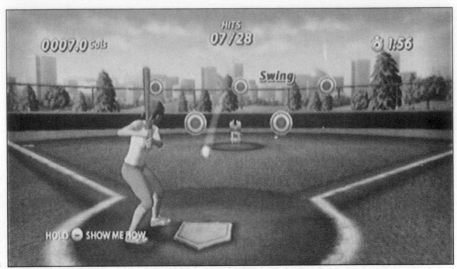

Figure 8-17: A typical Baseball screen, featuring Batting.

Catching

To catch, you need to move the Nunchuk in the direction that the ball is going as it travels toward you. To catch a ball on the left or right, swing the Nunchuk in that direction. To catch a pop fly or grounder, hold the Nunchuk up or down, respectively. After you've caught the ball, swing the Wii Remote to throw the ball toward the target. Swinging the Wii Remote harder for each throw provides a greater workout benefit.

Pitching

To pitch, swing the Wii Remote forward in a throwing motion. Swinging harder provides a greater workout benefit.

Wii Balance Board

When you use the Balance Board while playing Baseball, only how you catch the ball will change. When the sequence involving catching starts, you should be standing on the board with your feet shoulder-width apart and knees slightly bent. To catch a ball on the left, step off to the left and swing the Nunchuk to the left. Reverse for a ball on the right. After you've caught a ball, keep both feet on the board while you swing the Wii Remote to throw the ball toward the target.

Basketball

On the virtual basketball court, you perform two different activities involving the ball: passing and shooting. These are both considered upper body activities, though you can put more of your body into each pass and shot to greatly enhance the experience. You can also incorporate more lower body work and increase the challenge through the use of the Balance Board, though most of the movements are performed with the Wii Remote in your right hand and the Nunchuk in your left. An example of a typical Basketball screen is shown in Figure 8-18.

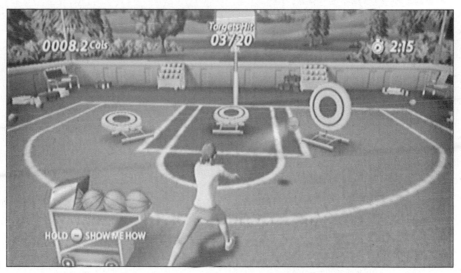

Figure 8-18:
A typical
Basketball
screen,
featuring
Passing.

Passing

To pass, first pick up a ball from the rack by swinging your arms to the left. When you have a ball, you're ready to pass. Push both hands forward with your elbows pointing out, using enough power to knock the target backward. Using more power for each pass provides a greater workout benefit.

Shooting

To shoot, first pick up a ball from the rack by swinging your arms to the left. After you have a ball, you're ready to shoot. Push both hands forward like you're shooting the ball toward the net. Using more power as you shoot provides a greater workout benefit and helps the ball reach the basket. The key to success here is getting into a good rhythm.

Wii Balance Board

When you use the Balance Board while playing Basketball, only passing the ball changes. When the sequence involving passing starts, you should be standing on the board with your feet shoulder-width apart and knees slightly bent. Pick up a ball off the rack by swinging your arms to the left. After you have a ball, aim at the target. To aim at the left target, take a step to the left with your foot. Reverse for the right target. To pass, push both hands forward with your elbows pointed out.

In-line Skating

Of all the sports activities in *EA Sports Active: Personal Trainer,* only In-line Skating (better known from the Nordica company trademark, Rollerblade) is designed to specifically target your lower body through a series of demanding squats and jumps. A lower impact effect can be achieved through use of the Balance Board. Even if you've never touched a pair of skates in your life, you'll be crouching for speed and jumping off ramps as you navigate around the virtual track, shown in Figure 8-19, in no time at all.

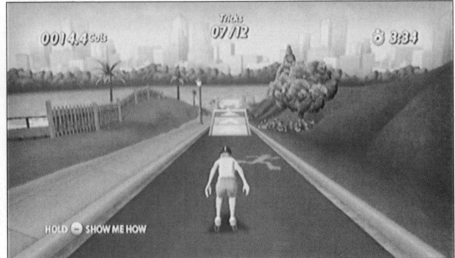

Figure 8-19:
A typical In-line Skating screen sans Balance Board.

To skate, you do a combination of squats and jumps. Place the Wii Remote in your right hand and the Nunchuk in the Leg Strap around your upper-right thigh. Stand with your feet shoulder-width apart and your knees slightly bent. Squatting will increase the speed with which you move down the track; thus, the lower you squat, the faster you will go, and the higher, the slower. When you come to the end of a ramp, jump up. Try to land softly and evenly with both feet and a slight bend in your knees to cushion the impact.

Wii Balance Board

When you use the Balance Board for In-line Skating, no jumping is involved, because doing so can damage the board. Stand on the board with your feet shoulder-width apart and your knees slightly bent. When you squat, you increase speed as you move down the track. The lower you squat, the faster you will go, and the higher, the slower. Instead of jumping, you'll be lifting your left or right leg in time to dodge hay bales on the track. If you fail to lift your leg over the bales, you will slow down.

Tennis

On the virtual tennis court, you work your upper body with volleys, ground-strokes, and overhead smashes. Most of the movements are performed with the Wii Remote in your right hand and the Nunchuk in your left, though you can incorporate more lower body work and increase the challenge through the use of the Balance Board. A typical Tennis screen is shown in Figure 8-20.

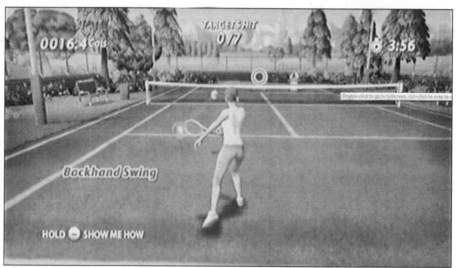

Figure 8-20: A typical Tennis screen, featuring the Backhand Swing.

Backhand

To do a backhand, quickly swing toward and through the ball. Rotate your shoulders and upper torso with the swing to get good full-body motion. Follow through by swinging across the body for the full range of the swing.

Backhand volley

For backhand volleys, raise the Wii Remote to about shoulder height. Bring your arms slightly across your body and behind. When the ball comes into position, quickly swing toward and through the ball. Your swings should be quick, short, and powerful.

Forehand

For a forehand shot, quickly swing forward through the ball. Rotate your shoulders and upper torso with the swing to get good full-body motion, following through by swinging across your body.

Forehand volley

When you're up close to the net, you volley. For the Forehand volley, raise the Wii Remote to about shoulder height. Bring your arms slightly back and behind you. When the ball comes into position, quickly swing through the ball.

Overhead Smash

When it's time to do overhead smashes, you see the ball launched high, as if it's going to go over your head. To hit these balls correctly, hold the Wii Remote slightly behind your head and over your shoulder. When the ball arrives, swing upward through its path, reaching as high as you can. Follow through completely to achieve a full range of motion. Your swinging hand should end on the opposite side of your body, below your shoulders, about the same height as your waist. Return to the ready position to prepare for the next ball.

Wii Balance Board

When you use the Balance Board while playing Tennis, only how you do backcourt forehands and backhands changes. When a sequence involving forehands or backhands starts, you should be standing on the board with your feet shoulder-width apart and knees slightly bent. If the ball is traveling to your right, step off the board with your right foot and swing the Wii Remote in a forehand stroke motion. After you've made your stroke, return your foot to the board. If the ball is traveling to your left, step off the board with your left foot and swing the Wii Remote in a backhand stroke motion. After you have made your stroke, return your foot to the board.

Volleyball

In Volleyball, you'll be on the virtual volleyball court targeting your upper body with bumping, setting, serving, and blocking, all without the risk of getting sand in your shorts. Although most of the movements are performed with the Wii Remote in your right hand and the Nunchuk in your left, you can put more of your body into each move and incorporate the Balance Board to enhance the experience, particularly for your lower body. A typical Volleyball screen is shown in Figure 8-21.

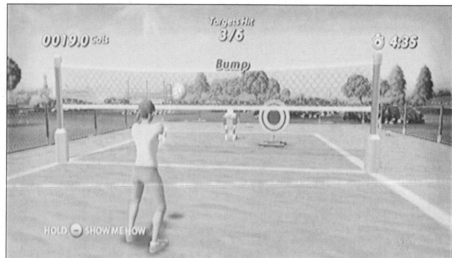

Figure 8-21:
A typical
Volleyball
screen,
featuring
Bumping.

Blocking

For blocking, bend your knees and keep your weight forward on the balls of your feet. Hold the Wii Remote and Nunchuk in front of your face. When the ball comes in range, jump into the air and push your hands up as high as you can to hit the ball back over the net.

Bumping

To bump, hold the Wii Remote and Nunchuk in front of you at waist height so they are touching. Bend your knees and keep your weight forward on the balls of your feet. When the ball is in range, straighten your legs and make a short swing upward with your arms.

Serving

To serve, keep your left hand at waist height and hold your right hand behind and to the right of your head. With your left hand, throw the ball up in the air by moving the Nunchuk sharply upward. As the ball starts to come back down, swing the Wii Remote downward to drive the ball over the net.

Setting

To set, hold your hands a few inches above and in front of your head so you can see them. Face your palms upward. When the ball is within range, push up with the Wii Remote and Nunchuk to set the ball.

Wii Balance Board

When you use the Balance Board while playing Volleyball, only how you do bumping and setting will change. When a sequence involving bumping or setting starts, you should be standing on the board with your feet shoulder-width apart and knees slightly bent. To bump, hold the Wii Remote and Nunchuk in front of you at waist height so they are touching. The ball will fall on either your left or right side. Step off the board to the side with the foot that the ball is falling toward and make a short swing upward to return the ball. To set, hold your hands a few inches above and in front of your head where you can see them. Face your palms upward. The ball will fall on either your left or right side. Step off the board in a lunge position to the side with the foot that the ball is falling toward and push up with the Wii Remote and Nunchuk to set the ball.

Chapter 9

Getting Active with the Routines

Despite countless claims made on magazine covers, late-night infomercials, and advertisements for supplements and fitness products, no "quick fix" exists when it comes to losing weight and getting in shape. Of course, exercise has numerous benefits, which you reap along the way, such as improved joint flexibility and reduced stress levels. Although patience and determination are essential in any quest to whip your body into the best shape possible, working out with routines that keep you engaged is equally important. When a routine stops being challenging, your muscles stop responding, leaving you at risk of throwing in the towel. EA Sports Active: Personal Trainer offers an abundance of workout regimens that contain a multitude of activities, including cardio, upper and lower body exercises, and sports-based drills, ensuring your workouts remain interesting and challenging. You also have the flexibility to create your own workouts or customize a preset routine.

In this chapter, we give you an overview of the *EA Sports Active: Personal Trainer* preset workouts. You also discover how you can create your own workouts or edit an existing one and learn how to assess your results and progress. We also provide you with a few routines that you can try. As you can see, this game has no shortage of workout options or activities from which you can choose. We begin by examining the preset routines.

Choosing From Preset Workouts

From the Main Menu, select Preset & Custom Workouts and then decide if you want to work out on your own or with a friend. If you choose to go solo, you have access to a wide range of workouts, including selections from the 30 Day Challenge. If you have previously selected the Wii Balance Board option for your profile, board-enabled exercises will replace certain exercises in the various preset workouts. The board option can be turned on or off from the Choose Workout screen by selecting the Wii Balance Board button in the lower-right corner, as shown in Figure 9-1. If you choose to work out with a friend, you will not be able to use the Balance Board, but a range of cooperative workouts is available in addition to selections from the 30 Day Challenge.

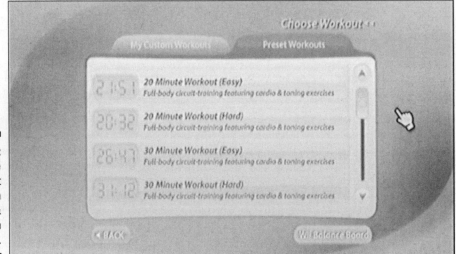

Figure 9-1:
The Choose
Workout
screen in
Preset &
Custom
Workouts.

In the typical exercise list, like the one shown in Figure 9-2, you can see the list of exercises under the Preset Workouts tab. Each workout option gives total time to completion if all exercises are selected and performed, what the workout is called, along with a Practice, Easy, Medium, or Hard descriptor to let you select your desired challenge level, and a slightly more detailed description, in red, of what the workout consists of.

After selecting the workout of your choice, the Today's Exercises screen appears, shown in Figure 9-2, which lists all the activities. The green check mark indicates that you will perform that exercise during the workout. If you see an exercise you'd rather not perform, or you wish to modify the time to completion or Calorie Target, you can click on an exercise to change the green check mark to a red x. Be sure you look at all the exercises in a particular workout by clicking through to the next page, as applicable, before clicking Continue.

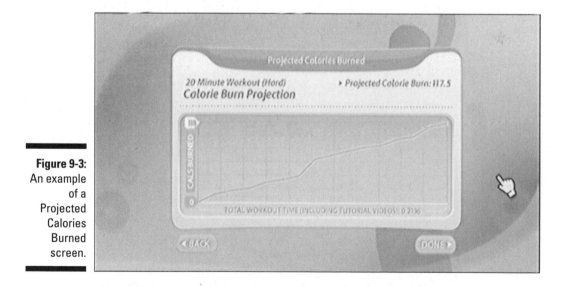

Figure 9-2:
A typical
Today's
Exercises
screen.

After you are satisfied with your preset workout selection and click Continue, you can see the Projected Calories Burned screen, an example of which is shown in Figure 9-3. The graph shows the logical progression of calories burned versus the time you spend working out, up until the workout's end, when you should reach the approximate final calorie projection.

Figure 9-3:
An example
of a
Projected
Calories
Burned
screen.

Clicking Done either brings you to the first tutorial video, which you can skip by pressing the A button, or to your first exercise. You're now ready to begin your workout!

Developing a Custom Workout

One of the most powerful features of *EA Sports Active: Personal Trainer* is its capability to allow you to create your own workout routines. Although there are enough preset workouts to keep you busy indefinitely, none of these may be tuned to your specific needs or preferences. Luckily, creating a custom workout in one of the four available slots is a relatively quick and intuitive process. It's also easy to edit a previously created custom workout or delete it entirely.

EA Sports Active: Personal Trainer gives you a wide range of exercises at three different skill levels in four different categories to choose from as you create your routine (for more on the exercises, refer to Chapter 8). Each skill level has differing difficulty and completion times and also provides a calorie burn estimate based on your bodyweight. Table 9-1 lists the Cardio exercises, Table 9-2 lists the Upper Body exercises, Table 9-3 lists the Lower Body exercises, and Table 9-4 lists the Sports exercises. Note that the Wii Balance Board exercises are not an option if you indicate you don't have a board or you choose to work out with a friend.

Table 9-1	Cardio Exercises		
Exercise	*Easy Time*	*Medium Time*	*Hard Time*
Heavy Bag	00:25	00:57	01:16
Targets & Heavy Bag 1	00:48	01:04	01:20
Targets & Heavy Bag 2	01:05	01:21	01:37
Targets & Heavy Bag 3	01:07	01:21	01:37
Targets & Heavy Bag 4	00:48	01:00	01:12
Targets & Heavy Bag 5	01:07	01:21	01:39
Wii Balance Board - Boxing - Targets & Heavy Bag	01:20	01:51	02:06
Targets 1	00:41	01:01	01:22
Targets 2	00:41	00:55	01:08
Targets 3	00:41	01:01	01:22
Targets 4	00:41	00:55	01:08
Boxing (Random Short)	00:25	00:57	01:16
Boxing (Random Medium)	00:41	01:01	01:22
Boxing (Random Long)	01:05	01:21	01:37
Dance Basic 1	00:52	01:13	01:47
Dance Basic 2	00:52	01:13	01:47

Exercise	Easy Time	Medium Time	Hard Time
Wii Balance Board – Dancing – Basic	00:52	01:13	01:47
Dance Intermediate 1	00:45	01:03	01:32
Dance Intermediate 2	00:45	01:03	01:32
Wii Balance Board – Dancing – Intermediate	00:45	01:03	01:32
Dance Fast 1	00:41	00:57	01:23
Dance Fast 2	00:41	00:57	01:23
Dance Fast 3	00:41	00:57	01:23
Dance Fast 4	00:41	00:57	01:23
Wii Balance Board – Dancing – Fast	00:41	00:57	01:23
Dance Fastest 1	00:34	00:47	01:09
Dance Fastest 2	00:34	00:47	01:09
Dancing (Random Basic)	00:45	01:03	01:32
Dancing (Random Intermediate)	00:34	00:47	01:09
Dancing (Random Pro)	00:34	00:47	01:09
Kick Ups (Short)	01:09	01:33	01:36
Kick Ups (Long)	03:06	03:30	03:13
Run & Walk (Short)	00:35	00:44	00:54
Run & Walk (Medium)	01:13	01:22	01:32
Run & Walk (Long)	01:51	02:01	02:10
Run (Short)	00:19	00:28	00:38
Run (Medium)	00:57	01:06	01:16
Run (Long)	01:35	01:44	01:54
Run (Very Long)	02:32	03:10	03:48
Run, Knees & Kick Ups 1	01:50	01:59	02:27
Run, Knees & Kick Ups 2	03:03	03:13	03:40
Walk & Run (Short)	00:35	00:44	00:54
Walk & Run (Medium)	01:13	01:22	01:32
Walk & Run (Long)	01:51	02:01	02:10
Track – Random (Easy)	00:19	00:28	00:38
Track – Random (Medium)	00:57	01:06	01:16
Track – Random (Hard)	03:06	03:30	03:13

Table 9-2	Upper Body Exercises		
Exercise	*Easy Time*	*Medium Time*	*Hard Time*
Alternating Bicep Curls	01:04	01:20	01:36
Alternating Cross Knee Punches	00:20	00:24	00:28
Alternating Shoulder Presses	00:48	01:12	01:36
Alternating Triceps Kickbacks	00:36	00:48	01:00
Bent Over Rows with Triceps Kickbacks	01:12	01:30	01:48
Bent Over Rows	00:32	00:40	00:48
Bicep Curls with Shoulder Presses	01:12	01:48	02:24
Bicep Curl with Upright Rows	01:28	02:12	02:56
Front Shoulder Raises	00:40	01:00	01:20
Lateral Shoulder Raises	00:32	00:48	01:04
Standing Twists	00:30	00:36	00:42
Upright Rows	00:48	01:12	01:36

Table 9-3	Lower Body Exercises		
Exercise	*Easy Time*	*Medium Time*	*Hard Time*
Alternating High Knee Reverse Lunges	01:00	01:24	02:00
Alternating Lunges	00:50	01:10	01:40
Alternating Side Lunges	01:00	01:24	02:00
Alternating Side Lunges with Toe Touches	01:20	01:52	02:40
Alternating Standing Knee Crunches	00:30	00:36	00:42
Jump Lunges	00:06	00:24	00:32
Jump Squats	00:24	00:36	00:48
Side to Side Jumps	00:24	00:32	00:40
Squat Holds	00:20	00:40	01:00
Squats	00:32	00:48	01:04
Squats with Calf Raises	01:04	01:36	02:08

Table 9-4	Sports Exercises		
Exercise	*Easy Time*	*Medium Time*	*Hard Time*
Passing 1	00:25	00:50	01:15
Passing 2	00:25	00:50	01:15
Wii Balance Board – Basketball	00:25	00:50	01:15
Shooting	00:38	01:16	01:54
Shooting & Passing 1	00:31	01:03	01:34
Shooting & Passing 2	00:44	01:03	01:34
Shooting & Passing 3	00:50	01:03	01:15
Basketball (Random Short)	00:38	01:16	01:54
Basketball (Random Medium)	00:31	01:03	01:34
Basketball (Random Long)	00:50	01:03	01:15
Inline Skating	00:51	01:03	02:03
Wii Balance Board – In-line Skating	00:51	01:03	02:03
Batting	00:39	01:01	01:20
Catching	00:47	01:02	01:18
Wii Balance Board – Baseball – Catching	00:47	01:02	01:18
Catching & Batting	00:47	01:10	01:27
Catching & Pitching	00:45	01:09	01:23
Pitch & Catch & Bat	00:46	01:14	01:27
Pitching	01:00	01:04	01:12
Pitching & Batting	01:02	01:21	01:28
Baseball (Random Short)	01:00	01:04	01:12
Baseball (Random Medium)	00:47	01:10	01:27
Baseball (Random Long)	00:46	01:14	01:27
Back Court	00:40	00:57	01:13
Wii Balance Board – Tennis	01:07	00:54	01:01
Back Court & Front Court	00:41	00:55	01:13
Back Court & Mid Court	00:45	01:10	01:45
Back, Front & Mid Court	00:51	00:57	01:34
Front Court	00:38	00:59	01:10
Front Court & Mid Court	00:42	01:06	01:34

(continued)

Table 9-4 *(continued)*

Exercise	Easy Time	Medium Time	Hard Time
Tennis (Random Short)	00:38	00:59	01:10
Tennis (Random Medium)	00:45	01:10	01:45
Tennis (Random Long)	00:51	00:57	01:34
Bump & Set	00:44	01:28	01:55
Wii Balance Board – Volleyball – Bump & Set	00:44	01:28	01:55
Bump, Set & Block	00:43	01:25	01:45
Serve & Bump	00:39	01:18	01:43
Serve, Bump & Set	00:41	01:16	01:28
Serve, Bump, Set & Block	00:55	01:28	01:59
Set & Block	00:41	01:22	01:42
Volleyball (Random Short)	00:41	01:22	01:42
Volleyball (Random Medium)	00:44	01:28	01:55
Volleyball (Random Long)	00:55	01:28	01:59

A harried schedule may make it easier for you to undertake two workouts in a day that are 15 minutes or less than one longer workout. If this is the case, consider creating mini routines for yourself that you can perform as time permits. Ideally, your mini routines focus on one half of your body, rather than including a mix of upper and lower body exercises.

Now try to create your first routine!

Creating your routine

Being able to create your own routines gives you a lot of flexibility with your workouts. It allows you to add variety to your workout, incorporate exercises that you enjoy or find challenging, or to target specific areas of your body. Follow these steps to create your own workout in *EA Sports Active: Personal Trainer:*

1. **From the Main Menu, select Preset & Custom Workouts and then decide if you want to work out on your own or with a friend, each of which has his or her own set of four custom workout slots.**

   If you select single player and have previously selected the Wii Balance Board option for your profile, board-enabled exercises will be available.

The board option also can be turned on or off from the Choose Workout screen by selecting the Wii Balance Board button in the lower-right corner (refer to Figure 9-1). If this is the first time you're creating a custom workout, you see the Create Your First Workout! button, which brings you to the Create My Workout screen, as shown in Figure 9-4.

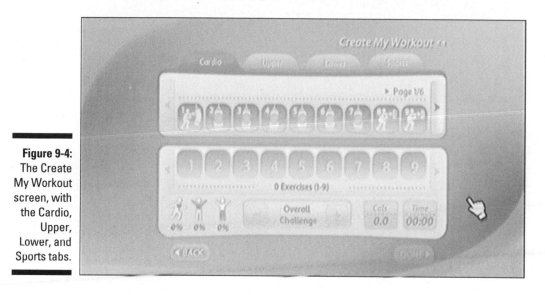

Figure 9-4:
The Create My Workout screen, with the Cardio, Upper, Lower, and Sports tabs.

2. **Add an exercise from one of the four onscreen tabs — Cardio, Upper, Lower, and Sports — by clicking on the exercise icon.**

   Refer to Tables 9-1 through 9-4 for the exercises that are available for each option. You can also drag and drop an exercise onto the list by clicking on its exercise icon and dragging it down to the list area while holding the A button, and then releasing it. When more than one exercise is in the list, you can drag and drop the exercises within the list to reorder them.

3. **After an exercise has been placed onto the list, you can change its default Medium difficulty by hovering the pointer over the icon until a selector appears, and either clicking the up arrow for Hard or the down arrow for Easy.**

   You can also change every exercise's difficulty on the list by pressing +, for more difficulty, or –, for less difficultly, in the Overall Challenge area toward the bottom of the screen. Clicking on an exercise in the list area removes it from the sequence. Each time you add a new exercise, the amount of projected calories burned and amount of time required to do the workout increase. You can also see the percentage focus on cardio, upper and lower body change via the indicators in the lower left. Generally speaking, the percentages only change if you mix in exercises from the different tabs.

Your body has finite recovery abilities, so a good rule is not to exceed a workout length of much more than 60 minutes. If you can work out longer than that, your intensity level probably needs to be increased.

4. **When you're happy with your exercise selection, the order, the total projected calories burned, the total workout time, and the body part mix, you're ready to save your new custom workout by selecting Done.**

   Your new workout populates the first available of the four save slots. After you choose a unique name and click OK, your workout will be saved and you'll be asked if you're ready to start your workout. It's now time to get to work!

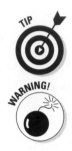

When all four save slots are filled, you must edit a workout — described in the next section — in order to make changes.

The four custom single player and the four custom two player workout slots are shared for all users of the *EA Sports Active: Personal Trainer* program. If you delete a custom workout using your profile, you delete that custom workout for everyone.

Editing your routine

After one or more of the four available workout slots are filled, you will have the capability to edit or delete these workouts. Clicking the red x allows you to delete, while clicking the blue pencil allows you to edit.

Follow these steps to edit a routine:

1. **If you generally like a workout routine you've created, but there is an exercise you don't want to perform on a certain day, simply click on the routine (not the pencil or x icons).**

   The Today's Exercises menu appears.

2. **Click on the green check mark for the exercise(s) you don't want to perform.**

   A red x appears next to these activities. If your routine includes more than eight exercises, be sure to scroll through all exercises by clicking the arrow on the right of the green check marks. When satisfied, click Continue. This shows you the projected calories burned, and once you click Done, your workout begins.

3. **If you want to add exercises, switch the order of the exercises, or permanently delete an activity from one of your custom routines, select the blue pencil icon for that routine.**

This opens the Create My Workout screen. To make your edits, follow the instructions as outlined in the "Creating Your Routine" section earlier in this chapter.

Trying these routines

Now that you know how to create a routine, you can try the three sample routines in Tables 9-5 through 9-7 that help tone your upper, lower, and total body, respectively, and assume you don't have access to a Wii Balance Board. These routines can help guide your thought process as you continue to build more of your own routines. Feel free to try these as-is or modify them for your specific needs or with your own ideas.

As we mention earlier, recovery is key. You want to train to failure, which is the point where you can no longer effectively perform exercises at maximum effort — but not beyond — as your body will have great difficulty repairing the muscle damage and rebuilding stronger for next time. If your body is constantly worn down, you can retard or even reverse your progress. For this reason, all the sample routines are well under 60 minutes. You want to train your body as hard as possible for as short of a time as possible and then spend the rest of the time eating right and resting for maximum gains. Particularly when first getting started, you are best served with one to two days of rest between every complete workout. If, for example, you work upper body on one day, you can take a break the next and then do lower body on the third. If you do a complete body workout, try taking two days off before your next strenuous activity. As you become more familiar with your body and how it responds, you can adjust these rest periods accordingly.

EA Sports Active: Personal Trainer does a good job of encouraging the use of exercise variety and targeting multiple body parts, but deviates slightly from the real-world standard of sets. A *rep,* or repetition, is merely the start to finish of an exercise motion. Multiple reps of an exercise motion comprise a set (for example, 8 to12 repetitions form a complete set). In lieu of multiple sets of a single exercise, *EA Sports Active: Personal Trainer* generally encourages doing a single set and moving on to the next exercise, perhaps returning to a particular exercise later on in the routine. The sample routines provide a more traditional approach of performing the same exercise for multiple sets. This traditional approach is easy to duplicate in the Create My Workout screen; simply add the same exercise to the list to match the desired number of sets. The advantage to multiple sets of the same exercise is simple — you're guaranteed to target the same exact muscle groups each time and really work them to failure. You also have a slightly lesser risk of injury as those same muscles should already be thoroughly warmed up.

Finally, in each of the sample routines, we begin with a warm-up, go through a logical body-part progression, do some cardio, and then end with a cooldown. By default, every exercise is set to Medium, but, depending upon your skill level, this can be adjusted up or down, which will also of course affect your total workout time and projected calories burn accordingly.

Stretching is not a warm-up. Stretching cold muscles can cause micro-tears. If you wish to stretch, do so carefully and only at the end of a workout after you're thoroughly warmed up.

Table 9-5	Upper Body Sample Routine		
Exercise	*Difficulty*	*Time*	*Function*
Targets & Heavy Bag 1	Easy	00:48	Warm Up
Alternating Bicep Curls	Medium	01:20	Exercise
Alternating Bicep Curls	Medium	01:20	Exercise
Alternating Shoulder Presses	Medium	01:12	Exercise
Alternating Shoulder Presses	Medium	01:12	Exercise
Alternating Shoulder Presses	Medium	01:12	Exercise
Upright Rows	Medium	01:12	Exercise
Upright Rows	Medium	01:12	Exercise
Alternating Triceps Kickbacks	Medium	00:48	Exercise
Alternating Triceps Kickbacks	Medium	00:48	Exercise
Bent Over Rows	Medium	00:40	Exercise
Bent Over Rows	Medium	00:40	Exercise
Bent Over Rows	Medium	00:40	Exercise
Standing Twists	Medium	00:36	Exercise
Standing Twists	Medium	00:36	Exercise
Targets & Heavy Bag 2	Medium	01:21	Exercise
Targets & Heavy Bag 3	Medium	01:21	Exercise
Targets & Heavy Bag 4	Medium	01:00	Exercise
Targets & Heavy Bag 5	Medium	01:21	Exercise
Run & Walk (Long)	Medium	02:01	Cardio
Run & Walk (Long)	Medium	02:01	Cardio
Walk & Run (Long)	Medium	02:01	Cardio
Walk & Run (Long)	Medium	02:01	Cardio
Shooting & Passing 1	Easy	00:31	Cool Down
Baseball (Random Medium)	Easy	01:10	Cool Down
TOTAL		28:41	

Table 9-6	Lower Body Sample Routine		
Exercise	*Difficulty*	*Time*	*Function*
Dance Basic 1	Easy	00:52	Warm Up
Squats	Medium	00:48	Exercise
Squats	Medium	00:48	Exercise
Squats	Medium	00:48	Exercise
Squats with Calf Raises	Medium	01:36	Exercise
Squats with Calf Raises	Medium	01:36	Exercise
Squats with Calf Raises	Medium	01:36	Exercise
Jump Squats	Medium	00:36	Exercise
Jump Squats	Medium	00:36	Exercise
Alternating Side Lunges	Medium	01:24	Exercise
Alternating Side Lunges with Toe Touches	Medium	01:52	Exercise
Alternating Side Lunges with Toe Touches	Medium	01:52	Exercise
Alternating Side Lunges with Toe Touches	Medium	01:52	Exercise
Side to Side Jumps	Medium	00:32	Exercise
Alternating Standing Knee Crunches	Medium	00:36	Exercise
Alternating Standing Knee Crunches	Medium	00:36	Exercise
Alternating Standing Knee Crunches	Medium	00:36	Exercise
Dance Basic 2	Medium	01:13	Cardio
Dance Intermediate 1	Medium	01:03	Cardio
Dance Intermediate 2	Medium	01:03	Cardio
Dance Fast 1	Medium	00:57	Cardio
Dance Fast 2	Medium	00:57	Cardio
In-line Skating	Easy	00:51	Cool Down
Volleyball (Random Long)	Easy	01:28	Cool Down
Tennis (Random Long)	Easy	00:51	Cool Down
TOTAL		26:26	

Table 9-7	Total Body Sample Routine		
Exercise	*Difficulty*	*Time*	*Function*
Boxing (Random Long)	Easy	01:05	Warm Up
Bicep Curls with Shoulder Presses	Medium	01:48	Exercise
Bicep Curls with Shoulder Presses	Medium	01:48	Exercise
Bent Over Rows with Triceps Kickbacks	Medium	01:30	Exercise
Bent Over Rows with Triceps Kickbacks	Medium	01:30	Exercise
Lateral Shoulder Raises	Medium	00:48	Exercise
Front Shoulder Raises	Medium	01:00	Exercise
Upright Rows	Medium	01:12	Exercise
Standing Twists	Medium	00:36	Exercise
Dance Basic 1	Easy	00:52	Warm Up
Squats	Medium	00:48	Exercise
Squats	Medium	00:48	Exercise
Squats	Medium	00:48	Exercise
Squats with Calf Raises	Medium	01:36	Exercise
Squats with Calf Raises	Medium	01:36	Exercise
Squats with Calf Raises	Medium	01:36	Exercise
Alternating Lunges	Medium	01:10	Exercise
Alternating High Knee Reverse Lunges	Medium	01:24	Exercise
Side to Side Jumps	Medium	00:32	Exercise
Side to Side Jumps	Medium	00:32	Exercise
Alternating Side Lunges with Toe Touches	Medium	01:52	Exercise
Alternating Side Lunges with Toe Touches	Medium	01:52	Exercise
Alternating Side Lunges with Toe Touches	Medium	01:52	Exercise
Track – Random (Hard)	Medium	01:06	Cardio
Track – Random (Medium)	Medium	01:06	Cardio
Track – Random (Easy)	Medium	00:28	Cardio
Walk & Run (Long)	Medium	02:01	Cardio

Exercise	Difficulty	Time	Function
Walk & Run (Medium)	Medium	01:22	Cardio
Walk & Run (Short)	Medium	00:44	Cardio
Runs, Knees & Kick Ups 1	Easy	01:59	Cardio
Baseball (Random Long)	Easy	00:46	Cool Down
TOTAL		39:34	

A regular, well-rounded workout regimen that targets all your core muscle groups is essential to obtaining results. Although it may be tempting to work certain body parts to the exclusion of others, this may leave your body looking off balance, especially after a desirable weight is reached. Further, it is impossible to spot reduce, meaning you can't target where your body will lose body fat. The human body tends to react systemically to stress, and you will lose weight from all areas of your body, including areas where you might like to retain your current shape. For instance, when many women lose weight, they find their breasts shrinking, much to their dismay. To keep your body looking balanced and counteract these effects, it is beneficial to work your whole body over a period of time, say every seven days. So even if you think you don't have to work your legs or chest, it's important for your continued progress to regularly include them in your workouts. Of course, you can place greater emphasis on certain muscles if you wish to build more strength in them.

Assessing Your Post-Workout Results

After you complete your workout, *EA Sports Active: Personal Trainer* provides you with your post-workout results, including Summary, Performance, and Goals screens. The first screen is the Summary screen, which lists the calories burned, workout time, and number of exercises completed in the left-hand column and provides trainer feedback in the right-hand column, as shown in Figure 9-5.

The following steps guide you through navigating your results:

1. **Click Next at the bottom right of the screen.**

   A Performance screen appears, which provides a graphical depiction of how many calories you burned (shown by the blue line) versus what was projected before your workout based on your bodyweight.

   See Figure 9-6 for an example of the Performance screen.

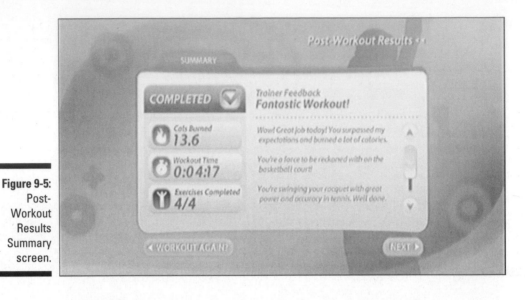

Figure 9-5:
Post-
Workout
Results
Summary
screen.

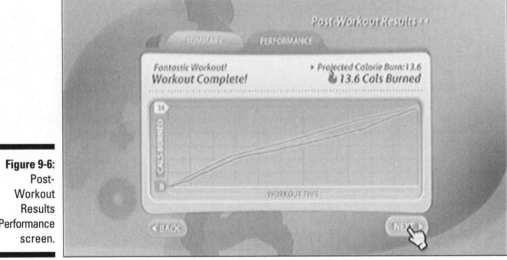

Figure 9-6:
Post-
Workout
Results
Performance
screen.

2. **Click Next at the bottom right of the screen again.**

   The Goals screen appears and shows you how far you've progressed toward your goals, provided you have a fitness profile and did not work out using a guest pass. See Figure 9-7 for an example of the Goals screen.

3. **Hover the cursor over each goal, including calories, hours, and workouts, to see what each of your current goal settings is and whether it has expired.**

   Turn to Chapter 7 for more on these goals and how to set them.

4. **Go back to any of the previous Post-Workout Results screens by clicking the Back button.**

   If you return to the Summary screen and click Back again, you will be brought back to the workout, which you can redo should you choose to do so.

5. **If you are done assessing your Post-Workout Results and do not want to repeat the regimen, continue to click Done.**

   You can also opt to see which trophies you've won by clicking Trophies at the bottom of the screen.

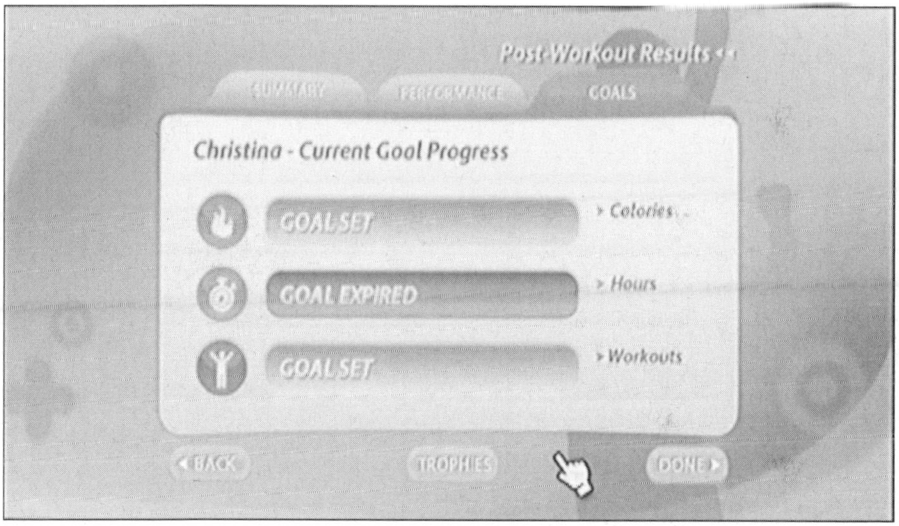

Figure 9-7:
Post-
Workout
Results
Goals
screen.

Although receiving trainer feedback and maintaining a record of your progress can be useful and fun, remember that no matter what the cold, hard data indicate, only you can truly judge your progress. If you feel like you got in a good workout, then you probably did. Little things such as getting an extra repetition or being able to do one more exercise than the last time, not to mention your clothing fitting better, are all very personal indicators that you're well on your way to achieving your goals. Although computer software can give you trophies and medals along the way, it can't give you the pride that comes from these physical accomplishments, which serve as the best measure of your progress.

Part III
Jillian Michaels Fitness Ultimatum 2010

The 5th Wave
By Rich Tennant

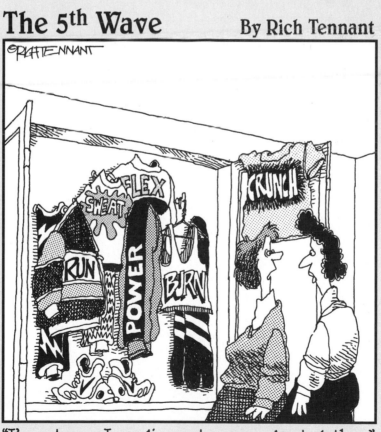

"I'm not sure I can live up to my workout clothes."

In this part . . .

While the two games featured in the first two parts of this book work hard to establish their brands, the game featured in this part take the comparatively easy way out by aligning with commercial juggernaut and fitness celebrity, Jillian Michaels. Of course, there's no easy way out for you as *Jillian Michaels Fitness Ultimatum 2010* is just as serious about working out as the other two games. Luckily, it's also as much fun. After being introduced to *Jillian Michaels Fitness Ultimatum 2010* and learning how to navigate through its various elements, you learn about the exercises and how to perform them. Finally, you find out how to work with the preset routines, as well as how to design your own. Who knows? You may be the next fitness celebrity getting in people's faces to motivate them!

Chapter 10

Getting Started

. . . .

In This Chapter

▶ Finding out about the program

▶ Creating a profile

▶ Navigating the Island Hub

. . . .

Majesco's *Jillian Michaels Fitness Ultimatum 2009,* released in the United States on October 21, 2008, was advertised as the first game of its type to "combine a celebrity fitness trainer with the Wii and innovative Wii Balance Board accessory to offer you a fun and entertaining way to get fit." Although the first part of that statement is factually correct and no doubt helped the game sell over 500,000 copies in its first five months alone, its actual execution left much to be desired. From lackluster visuals to a confusing menu system to poor motion control tracking, *Jillian Michaels Fitness Ultimatum 2009* disappointed many of *The Biggest Loser* star's legion of fans. Luckily, Majesco quickly went back to the drawing board and enlisted a new developer for *Jillian Michaels Fitness Ultimatum 2010,* which was released on October 6, 2009, and addressed many of the first game's shortcomings by greatly simplifying the experience. Although the 2009 version supports multiple control schemes and multiplayer functionality, 2010 supports just a single Wii Remote and optional Balance Board, and drops multiplayer entirely, focusing instead on a quality one-on-one experience with the virtual fitness celebrity. Speaking of Jillian Michaels, her digital avatar has never looked better and the rest of the game's visuals have received a similar boost. A new surprise feature makes the 2010 version accessible to more people — the game now can be played in Spanish!

This chapter provides you with all you need to know to get started using *Jillian Michaels Fitness Ultimatum 2010.* You find out about the game's features, create a profile, navigate the menus, personalize your experience, and more, as we team up with Jillian Michaels to guide you on your fitness adventure.

Introducing Jillian Michaels Fitness Ultimatum 2010

With motion-captured movements, fitness routines, and audio from Jillian Michaels herself, *Jillian Michaels Fitness Ultimatum 2010* makes good use of its celebrity branding, including having her digital avatar present for one-on-one training throughout the game. You can work out in one of ten different Pacific island locations with 18 unique exercises, described in Chapter 11, that really put your strength and cardiovascular system to the test. A Resolutions mode features a customizable training calendar that lets you plan exercise routines for up to six months (see Chapter 12). Adjustable difficulty levels and a focus on safely warming up and cooling down help round out the *Jillian Michaels Fitness Ultimatum 2010* experience. Now that you know what's in store for you with the game, you can begin your journey not in the negative as the biggest loser, but in the positive as the biggest winner. You can do it!

Registering Your Information

After starting the game, you are presented with a brief video introduction from Jillian Michaels and then immediately taken to the Registration Menu. At the Registration Menu, you have the choice of one of three options: New Profile, Existing Profile, or Guest, the last of which offers access to all of the game's features except for Resolutions, but does not save any data. Whenever you select any of the three options, you are asked if you have a Wii Balance Board. If you do have a Balance Board and have not already synced it with your Wii, please refer to Chapter 1 for setup information; otherwise, power it on and select Yes when prompted. You are guided through a brief calibration process, including a weigh-in. Note that the weigh-in does not ask you for the weight of your clothes, so keep that in mind when you see the number on the Profile screen.

Even if you answer No to having a Balance Board, you can still perform the Balance Board activities without tracking, by mirroring the movements of Jillian's avatar.

When entering a New Profile, you are asked for the following information: Name, Age, Height, Weight, and Gender. Using your Wii Remote, enter the requested information by clicking on the appropriate label with the A button. Click DEL to erase any mistakes, press your Wii Remote's B button to exit the data entry without saving, or click Enter when you're happy and done with your input. Note that there is an eight-character limit for names in the program, so if you have a long first name like one of the authors of this book, you need to figure out an alternative. If you have a Balance Board, you do not need to manually enter your weight.

The only information you need to enter when creating a New Profile before proceeding is your name, but it's better if you take the time to enter everything else as well. Of course, you can always go to Edit My Profile under My Info at any time to change any of the information, except for your name, which is permanent unless you erase your entire profile.

There are only four available profile slots, so if you try to create a New Profile with all four slots already taken, you will be given the option of erasing an existing profile. This is also the only way you can remove a profile once it has been created, so it pays to create carefully in the first place!

Just like *EA Sports Active: Personal Trainer, Jillian Michaels Fitness Ultimatum 2010* does not keep track of your birthday, so be sure to update your age in the game every time your age changes to ensure accurate tracking.

Navigating the Island Hub

After creating a New Profile, choosing an Existing Profile, or signing in as a Guest, you are presented with the Island Hub, shown in Figure 10-1, and described in detail in the following sections.

Press B at any time on your Wii Remote to go back to the preceding screen.

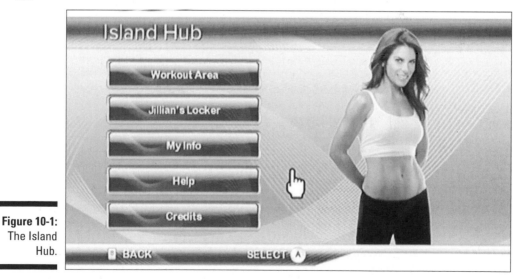

Figure 10-1:
The Island
Hub.

The Workout Area

The Workout Area consists of Island Overview, Single Exercise, Circuit Training, and Resolutions, as shown in Figure 10-2. The following list describes each part.

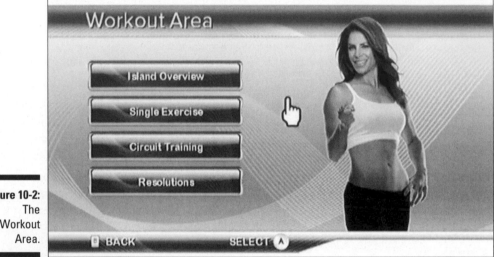

Figure 10-2:
The
Workout
Area.

✔ **Island Overview:** The game picks a random exercise at a predetermined difficulty level for you once you select one of the available locations: Cascade, Pier, Desert, Sand Dunes, Marshland, Rock, Jungle, Hilltop, Beach Landing, or Random. As opposed to Single Exercise, this area is best for when you really aren't sure what you feel like doing or want a surprise.

✔ **Single Exercise:** This area allows you to specify all of the details you couldn't in the Island Overview. You get to choose your exercise, the number of repetitions, the location you want to work out in, and the background music. For more information on this area, refer to Chapter 11.

✔ **Circuit Training:** Choose between one of Jillian's Circuits that focuses on a particular area of your body, or one of your own, either already created or built on the spot. For more on Circuit Training, turn to Chapter 12.

✔ **Resolutions:** This area enables you to create a custom workout schedule for up to six months, or you can select a premade schedule provided by Jillian Michaels. For more on Resolutions, see Chapter 11.

Jillian's Locker

Enter Jillian's Locker if you are in the mood to change her avatar's outfit, you want basic diet or exercise tips, or you are in need of some encouragement. Tips include nuggets such as "go through your kitchen and throw out all the junk food and processed garbage immediately — you can't eat it if it's not there" and "exercise is the architect, and recovery is the builder. Your muscles need adequate recovery time to rebuild and get stronger." While Jillian is tough on *The Biggest Loser* and doesn't tolerate slip-ups, the tips here acknowledge that it can be tough to always make healthy choices, and they serve to encourage you even through times of weakness. As you use the program, more tips will become unlocked. Let's briefly explore the three options in this area:

- **Outfits:** Outfits allows you to choose between three workout outfits, each with three different color combinations (though two of them look virtually identical), for Jillian to wear during the game. You can rotate Jillian's avatar by pressing left and right on the D pad or by clicking on the blue arrows that appear on either side of her. You can also zoom in on her upper body by pressing up and down on the D pad. Onscreen icons indicate the D-pad movements for zooming in and rotating, but the labels for these are transposed, indicating you press up and down to rotate the avatar and left and right to zoom in, but this is incorrect.

- **Diet Tips:** Diet Tips enables you to view tips covering Diet Goals, Food, and Eating Out by clicking each of their respective tabs on the screen. After you select the tab you want, you can read through each of the tips in these categories by clicking the Previous and Next buttons on the bottom of the screen. More diet tips become unlocked as you use the program.

- **Exercise Tips:** Exercise Tips allows you to view tips covering exercise Goals, Time, and Mind, each of which has its own tab. Although none of this information is presented in a particularly compelling manner, the tips themselves are sound. You can read through the tips contained under each of these tabs by selecting the one you want, and then clicking the Previous and Next buttons on the bottom of the screen. As you continue to use the program, more tips become unlocked.

My Info

As the name implies, this area is all about you. Here you can modify and view your various in-game settings, including your profile, stats, options, and resolutions. The following list examines each setting more closely.

- ✔ **Edit My Profile:** Allows you to see your Name and change your Age, Height, Weight, and Gender as necessary.

- ✔ **My Stats:** View your overall achievements and weight loss (or gain) to date.

- ✔ **My Options:** Consists of two options, Sound and Troubleshoot Mode. Sound allows you to change the volume for Voice, Music, and Environment so that you can get the most pleasing mix. Troubleshoot Mode lets you redo the calibration for your Wii Balance Board to verify that it is working correctly.

- ✔ **My Resolution:** View your Resolutions Calendar. For more on Resolutions, see Chapter 11.

Help

You can use two options here — Exercise Help and Scoring Help. Select Exercise Help to get a personal explanation from Jillian Michaels for every available Wii Remote and Balance Board exercise and Scoring Help to view an explanation of how scoring works.

Credits

Select this option to see who had a hand in making *Jillian Michaels Fitness Ultimatum 2010.*

Chapter 11

Tackling the Exercises

A good Wii fitness game provides quality exercises, and all of the games we cover in this book do this. What distinguishes *Jillian Michaels Fitness Ultimatum 2010* from the rest is its use of explosive movements. Performing exercises explosively can increase your strength and heart rate as well as facilitate greater fat loss by helping to push your body beyond its usual abilities. Although ballistic motions can have great benefit, explosive exercises always need to be performed with great care because they can increase your risk of injury, particularly if you have sloppy form. Although it's important to remain aware of and in control of your body at all times, it's especially critical when performing explosive exercises such as those included in *Jillian Michaels Fitness Ultimatum 2010*.

In this chapter, we discuss how your exercise performance is scored, review how you can customize the Single Exercise workout area, and provide an overview of the individual exercises themselves and how to perform them. Exercises are organized based on whether they use the Wii Remote or Balance Board or whether they are intended for cooling down. Although you can power through explosive exercises, be sure to perform them at your own pace.

Examining Exercise Tracking and Scoring

Exercises use either the Wii Remote or the Balance Board, as outlined in Table 11-1, to track your movements by checking predetermined positions of the exercises against those of your Wii Remote or detecting weight shifts on your Balance Board. Your exercise performance — except when warming up and cooling down — is tracked onscreen by using the game's Pulse Bar.

The Pulse Bar is separated into four quadrants, each of which appears based on the motion of the exercise, then changes color to green, red, or yellow depending upon your timing while performing an exercise repetition.

If you do not have a Wii Balance Board, you can still perform the exercises, but your movements will not be tracked and you will be given a default 80 percent of the possible points. Remember, Wii fitness is about maximizing your health, not maximizing your points, so be sure to work out intensely and with good form, even when you aren't being tracked.

One exercise repetition can be worth a maximum of ten points if it is done correctly in time with Jillian's onscreen avatar. If you can't keep pace with Jillian, you can still get some of the points by getting your Pulse Bar to turn yellow. If you do the exercise completely incorrectly, the Pulse Bar flashes red and no points will be awarded.

Table 11-1	The Exercises	
Exercise	*Accessory*	*Body Part(s) Trained*
Back Kick	Wii Remote	Glutes, Shoulders, Lower Back
Bicycle	Balance Board	Abdominals
Boat Pose	Balance Board	Abdominals
Closed Push-Up	Balance Board	Chest, Triceps, Shoulders, Abdominals, Core
Crunch	Balance Board	Abdominals
Hip Twist	Wii Remote	Abdominals, Obliques
Jumping Jack	Wii Remote	Cardiovascular System
Lunge Kick	Balance Board	Quadriceps, Glutes, Abdominals
Oblique	Wii Remote	Obliques
Pelvic Thrust	Balance Board	Glutes, Abdominals
Push-Up	Balance Board	Chest, Triceps, Shoulders
Running	Wii Remote	Cardiovascular System
Side Lunge	Wii Remote	Quadriceps, Glutes
Side Plank	Balance Board	Core
Sledge Swing	Wii Remote	Quadriceps, Glutes, Anterior Deltoids

Exercise	Accessory	Body Part(s) Trained
Squat Jacks	Wii Remote	Cardiovascular System, Quadriceps, Glutes
Swing Kick	Balance Board	Glutes, Adductors
Water Pump	Wii Remote	Quadriceps, Glutes, Shoulders, Trapezius

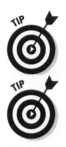

If you want to change your point of view during any of the exercises, use the D-Pad on your Wii Remote. Pushing up zooms in, pushing down zooms out, and pressing left or right moves the camera in either direction, respectively.

You can press + on your Wii Remote at any time during an exercise in a circuit to bring up the Pause menu, where you have the choice of continuing or quitting the exercise entirely.

Customizing the Single Exercise Workout Area

To customize individual exercises, select the Single Exercise option after selecting Workout Area from the Island Hub main menu. Figure 11-1 shows four tabs: Exercise, Location, Music, and Done. We describe each tab in the following list.

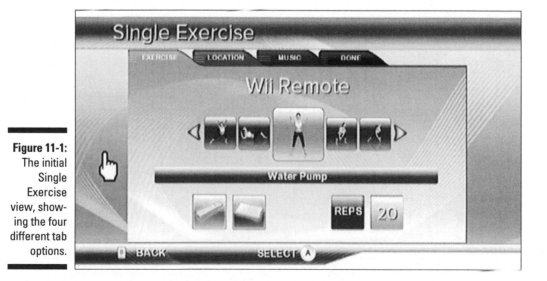

Figure 11-1: The initial Single Exercise view, showing the four different tab options.

✔ **Exercise tab:** Select the Wii Remote or Wii Balance Board icon on the lower left of the screen to select between Wii Remote and Balance Board exercises. Click on the blue Reps icon to change the number of repetitions required to complete the exercise. You can choose from Easy, Medium, and Hard ranges of repetitions, each with its own minimum and maximum thresholds.

✔ **Location tab:** Choose from Beach Landing, Cascade, Desert, Hilltop, Jungle, Marshland, Pier, Rock, Sand Dunes, and Random, the last of which is indicated by the question mark icon.

✔ **Music tab:** Choose from 20 different music selections, plus a random option, which is indicated by the question mark icon. You can also choose to preview your music selection to help guide your decision.

✔ **Done tab:** This is the last step needed for you to perform the exercise using your customizations. Here you see a summary of your selections, and after you are satisfied with them, click the Start button to begin the exercise.

Working Out with Wii Remote Exercises

Of the 18 available exercises, 9 use the Wii Remote. Although these include both upper and lower body strength movements and cardiovascular exercises, each one requires you to hold the Wii Remote in one of your hands. The last thing we want is for your TV screen or other prized possession to go Kaboom! while you are working out, so be sure to use the Wii Remote's wrist strap to prevent the Wii Remote from flying out of your hand while you are performing these explosive exercises.

Water Pump

As you likely guessed, Water Pump simulates the activity of manually pumping water. This exercise works the tops of your upper thighs (quadriceps) and buttocks (glutes) through its squatting motion, while also targeting your shoulder and neck (trapezius) muscles through its upright rowing motion. Follow these steps to try this exercise:

1. **Stand with your feet pointing forward and shoulder width apart. Raise your arms up as if you were grabbing a pump handle — in this case your Wii Remote — making sure that your elbows remain above your hands, as shown in Figure 11-2.**

   Keep your torso upright and your eyes focused on a point in front of you, chin up.

2. **Drop into a squat while pushing down the Wii Remote, as if you were pushing on a pump handle.**

   As you squat, make sure that your knees do not travel over your toes.

3. **Slowly come up out of the squat as you return your arms to their starting position.**

4. **Repeat according to the onscreen instructions.**

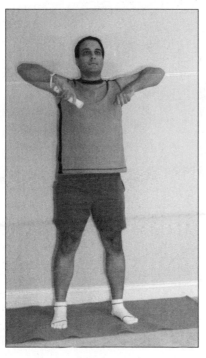

Figure 11-2:
The start position of the Water Pump.

Sledge Swing

The Sledge Swing primarily works the tops of your upper thighs and buttocks through its squatting motion as well as the front of your shoulders (anterior deltoid) through its front raise motion. This exercise mimics swinging a sledge hammer. Now, get to building that power with these steps:

1. **Hold your Wii Remote in both hands, fingers crossed, as if you were grasping the handle of a sledge hammer.**

2. **Stand, legs straight, with your feet just beyond shoulder width apart and toes pointing forward.**

3. While still grasping your Wii Remote, bring your arms to your side and then up and over your head. Exhale sharply as you swing your Wii Remote down to the floor between your legs as you squat, being sure not to round your back, as shown in Figure 11-3.

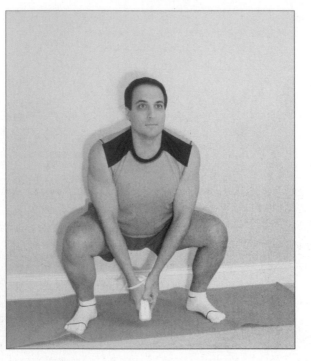

Figure 11-3: The bottom position of the Sledge Swing.

4. Bring the Wii Remote up and around to your other side as you inhale. Exhale sharply as you swing your Wii Remote down to the floor between your legs as you squat.

5. Repeat according to the onscreen instructions.

Hip Twist

Not to be confused with the Hip Twist in pilates that involves pivoting your lower body, the *Jillian Michaels Fitness Ultimatum 2010* version uses a different angle, primarily working your stomach muscles, particularly those at the side of your waist. Start chiseling your midsection by following these steps:

1. Hold your Wii Remote in your right hand with both arms extended out to each side and parallel to the floor.

2. Stand with your feet farther than hip width apart, with your back straight and head looking forward.

3. As you exhale, swing your right hand down to your left foot as you bend your left knee. Touch your foot and then return to the starting position. Without stopping, inhale as you take your left hand down to your right foot as you bend your right knee and return to the standing position.

4. Repeat according to the onscreen instructions.

Oblique

The obliques are the muscles at the sides of your waist. The aptly named Oblique exercise primarily targets these muscles, while also working the rest of your stomach. If you desire six-pack abdominals, working the obliques is imperative to completing the look. To develop obliques magnifique, follow these steps:

1. Lay on your back with your knees bent and feet flat on the floor, spread about a foot apart.

2. Hold your Wii Remote behind your head with the buttons facing the back of your head and the top of the controller pointing away from you.

    Your elbows should be flat on the ground.

3. Use your stomach muscles to curl your body upward while you bring one elbow toward the opposite knee and exhale as you go.

    You can only go up about halfway because your opposite elbow should remain on the ground.

4. Slowly return back down to the starting position and inhale as you go.

5. Repeat the motion for the opposite side and continue according to the onscreen instructions.

Side Lunge

Lunges are great for gaining definition in your legs and banishing thigh jiggle. The side lunge primarily works the tops of your upper thighs and buttocks. Follow these steps to perform this exercise:

1. Hold your Wii Remote in either hand and stand with your feet together and arms at your sides.

2. Keep your feet pointed forward and take a step to the side (lunge) with one leg, bending at your hip until your thigh is parallel to the floor.

Your step knee should be over your ankle while your opposite leg is kept straight with your foot flat on the ground. As you take the step to the side, bring your arms to eye level, parallel to the floor, and point the Wii Remote forward with each lunge.

3. **Return to the starting position and repeat the same motion for your other side.**

Continue according to the onscreen instructions.

Back Kick

The Back Kick primarily works your buttocks, with a secondary focus on your shoulders and lower back. Get those buns of steel by following these steps:

1. **Hold your Wii Remote in either hand, stand with your feet about shoulder width apart, elbows bent, and hands close to your chest.**

2. **Kick your right foot out behind you as you thrust both arms forward at eye level and bend at the waist so your body is parallel to the ground, as shown in Figure 11-4.**

3. **Bring your hands back toward your chest as you lower your leg back to the floor and straighten to a standing position.**

4. **Switch sides and repeat according to the onscreen instructions.**

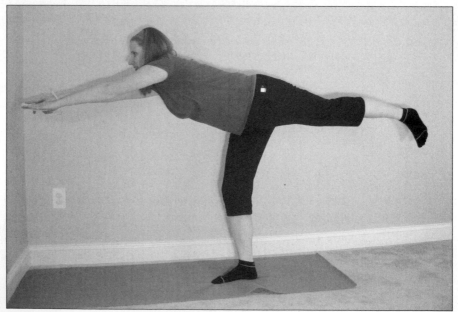

Figure 11-4:
The apex of the Back Kick.

Jumping Jack

Jumping Jacks do more than bring back memories of high school gym class. They also are great at targeting your cardiovascular system. While you likely do not need an overview of how to perform this activity, it is our job to instruct you, so here we go:

1. **Hold your Wii Remote in either hand and point it at the ground.**

2. **Stand with your feet together, back straight, and your arms at your side.**

3. **Jump, bringing your arms over your head and landing with your feet about shoulder width apart and your Wii Remote pointed at the ceiling.**

4. **Jump again and return to the starting position.**

5. **Repeat according to the onscreen instructions.**

Squat Jacks

As a fusion of the Jumping Jack and squats, Squat Jacks primarily target your cardiovascular system, the tops of your upper thighs, and your buttocks. These are great for combating cellulite, which is a common problem for women and also affects some men. Wage war on cellulite while gaining lower body strength by following these steps:

1. **Stand straight with your arms at your sides, Wii Remote pointed at the ground in either hand, and feet shoulder width apart.**

2. **Jump, bringing your arms over your head, landing in a squat position with your knees bent at 45 degrees and your Wii Remote pointed at the ceiling.**

3. **Using your legs and buttocks, push yourself back to the starting position.**

4. **Repeat according to the onscreen instructions.**

Running

Running targets your cardiovascular system and is a great way to build endurance. Although *Wii Fit Plus* and *EA Sports Active: Personal Trainer* offer running activities, this is your chance to go for a jog on a lush Pacific island without having to buy a plane ticket. Follow these steps to go for a run using *Jillian Michaels Fitness Ultimatum 2010:*

1. **Hold the Wii Remote in either hand.**

2. **Jog in place while pumping your arms up and down, making sure with each step your knees rise up high and you land softly.**

   Continue until time expires.

Performing Wii Balance Board Exercises

The following nine exercises use your Wii Balance Board and feature a range of strength-based movements. Many of these exercises require you to get on the floor.

Even if you don't have a Wii Balance Board, you can still perform the Balance Board exercises without tracking, by mirroring Jillian's avatar.

Boat Pose

The Boat Pose is a yoga pose that is referred to by yogis as Navasana. This pose, which primarily targets your stomach muscles, is similar to *Wii Fit Plus*'s Grounded V, which we cover in Chapter 3. Here is how you do the pose:

1. **Lay flat on your back, arms at your side, with the back of your heels on your Balance Board.**

2. **Lift your hands about six inches above the floor with your palms facing in as you bring your legs and upper body together in a "V" position.**

3. **In a controlled manner, slowly lay back down to assume the starting position.**

   For maximum effect, do not bend your arms or knees. Repeat per the onscreen instructions.

Crunch

Crunches are sometimes referred to as curl-ups, and they are one of the most common exercises to target the stomach muscles. While these are thought to be gentler on your back than traditional sit-ups, they can still be taxing on the spine. If you have back problems, you may opt to avoid these, as there are many other exercises that are great at working your abdominals. If you want to start crunching, follow these steps:

1. **Sit on the floor with your Balance Board behind you.**

2. **Lay back so that your head rests in the center of your Balance Board.**

3. Place your feet flat on the ground with your knees about a foot apart.

4. Interlock your hands behind your head, elbows wide apart and thumbs behind your ears.

5. Take a deep breath and exhale as you curl up and forward using just your stomach muscles until your shoulder blades are off the floor. Your hands are only there to support your head, not lift it. Hold at the top position for a brief moment, exhale, and lower yourself back down to the floor in a controlled manner.

6. Repeat for the indicated number of repetitions.

Swing Kick

An exercise inspired by martial arts, the Swing Kick primarily work your buttocks and the inside part of your upper thighs (adductors). Follow these steps to build powerful legs that you can use to protect yourself should you ever find yourself accosted in a dark alley:

1. Stand in front of your Balance Board with your feet about shoulder width apart.

2. Bring your hands up and hold them in a midpoint position for balance.

3. Swing your left leg up and over in a powerful motion so you end up touching the right side of your Balance Board, as shown in Figure 11-5.

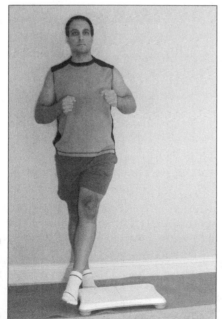

Figure 11-5:
Mid-point
for the
Swing Kick.

4. Swing your left leg back up and over to return to the starting position.

5. When prompted, switch sides, and repeat with your right leg touching the left side of your Balance Board.

6. Repeat for each side as indicated on the screen.

Lunge Kick

The Lunge Kick primarily works the tops of your upper thighs, your buttocks, and your stomach muscles. This exercise is another great one to add to your cellulite-busting repertoire. Follow these steps to perform the exercise:

1. Stand on your Balance Board with your feet spread evenly apart and your arms at your side.

2. Extend your right leg back, off of your Balance Board, until your left leg bends 90 degrees, as you inhale and swing both arms forward with your palms down until your arms are fully extended and parallel to the floor.

3. Bring your right leg forward and thrust your knee up at the ceiling as you exhale and move your arms down to your sides, back to the start position.

4. Repeat the same steps with your other leg and continue alternating according to the onscreen instructions.

Bicycle

Bicycles work your stomach muscles, with a particular focus on the rectus abdominis muscles. These are the muscles that give you that much sought after six-pack, provided you also watch your diet. To start working on those washboard abs, follow these steps:

1. Place the backs of your thighs across your Balance Board until your buttocks is resting against the edge.

2. Lay back, flat on the floor, and put your arms at your sides with your palms facing in.

3. Raise your right knee toward your chest as far as you can and then bring it back down so that the back of it touches your Balance Board. As you lower your right leg, raise your left knee to your chest.

4. Repeat in a continuous motion according to the onscreen instructions.

Side Plank

Just like *Wii Fit Plus*'s Plank, discussed in Chapter 3, *Jillian Michaels Fitness Ultimatum 2010*'s Side Plank works your core muscles, builds upper body strength, and requires quite a bit of balance. Follow these steps to perform the exercise:

1. **Place your hands on your Balance Board with your body in a standard push-up position, described later in this chapter and shown in Figure 11-6, as your starting point.**

2. **While balancing on your left arm, slowly roll your body back as your right arm extends to the ceiling.**

3. **Bring your right arm back down to the starting position and shift your weight to this side as you repeat the motion with your left arm.**

4. **Continue alternating sides according to the onscreen instructions.**

Pelvic Thrust

The Pelvic Thrust primarily works your buttocks, with secondary emphasis on your stomach muscles. This exercise helps you gain definition in your rear. Here is how you perform the exercise:

1. **Place your Balance Board on the floor and sit your buttocks on top of it in the center. Lightly grasp the sides of your Balance Board.**

2. **Bend your legs, keeping your feet flat on the ground as you lean back into the starting position.**

3. **Lift your buttocks as high as you can off the Balance Board.**

4. **Lower your buttocks back down to the starting position, touching the Balance Board.**

5. **Repeat according to the onscreen instructions.**

Push-Up

The Push-Up in *Jillian Michaels Fitness Ultimatum 2010* works the same chest, shoulder, and arm muscles as *Wii Fit Plus*'s version, which is discussed in Chapter 3. It is also good at strengthening your stomach muscles if you keep your back straight and use your abs as a brace to keep your body locked in place. Follow these steps to perform the exercise:

1. **Place your hands just outside the edges of your Balance Board so that you're straddling it with your arms.**

2. **Extend your lower body behind you. Raise your arms to full extension and rise up on the balls of your feet, being sure to keep your upper and lower body straight and in line throughout the movement, as shown in Figure 11-6.**

3. **Lower your body down by bending your arms until your chest touches the Balance Board, and then push back up to the starting position.**

4. **Repeat according to the onscreen instructions.**

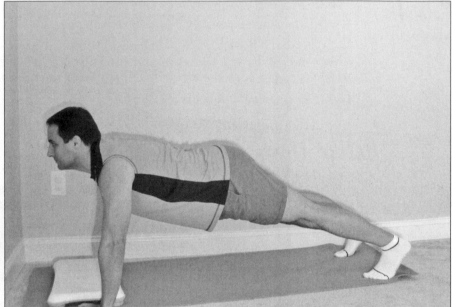

Figure 11-6:
The start position for the Push-Up.

Closed Push-Up

Much like the Push-Up, the Closed Push-Up works you chest, shoulder, and arm muscles, with additional emphasis on your stomach muscles and overall core. This exercise also requires a great deal of balance. Follow these steps to perform the Closed Push-Up:

1. **Place your hands on your Balance Board with your body in a standard Push-Up position, as described for Push-Ups and shown in Figure 11-6, as your starting point.**

2. **Bend your arms to touch your chest to your Balance Board.**

3. **At the top of the Push-Up, rotate your body to the right, lifting your right hand off the ground as your left knee swings up to meet your right hand.**

4. **Return to the starting position and repeat the same motions for your other side.**

5. **Repeat according to the onscreen instructions.**

Cooling Down Exercises

Although the exercises described earlier are available at any time, the two cool-down exercises we describe in the following sections are only available during Circuit Training, which is described in Chapter 12. Because it is unnecessary to track a cool down, neither exercise makes use of the Wii Remote or the Balance Board.

Knees to Chest

Knees to Chest shares many similarities with the Bicycle, except instead of actively moving your legs, you're focusing on holding various positions and stretching. Follow Jillian's avatar for additional variations while performing this movement. Here is how to perform the basic Knees to Chest:

1. **Lay down flat on your back.**

2. **Bring your knees to your chest.**

3. **Grab one knee with the same side arm and lower the other leg. Switch legs only when Jillian's avatar does so.**

Lunge Stretch

The Lunge Stretch is a less active form of the regular Lunge, where once you are in the bottom position, you concentrate on holding the pose and stretching. You can perform this stretch many ways; we describe one method. Similarly, you can also follow along with the variations that Jillian's avatar employs. Remember, the point of a cool down is to wind down, so don't overdo it!

1. **Stand up straight, with your feet pointing forward and just under shoulder width apart.**

2. **Move your right leg back, placing your lower leg and knee on the floor as you extend your left leg out in front of you, touching your hands to the floor as you keep your head up.**

   To intensify the stretch, lower your head.

3. **Hold this position until Jillian's avatar switches positions, and then reverse the sequence for the other side of your body.**

Chapter 12

Running through the Routines

In This Chapter
▶ Examining Circuit Training
▶ Establishing Resolutions

Sticking with an exercise routine is among the biggest challenges facing people looking to get healthier. Whether it's boredom, lack of motivation, or lack of results, any number of factors go into a person losing momentum and lacking the motivation to keep working out. A game, such as *Jillian Michaels Fitness Ultimatum 2010,* is the next best thing to having a live fitness celebrity get on your case and keep you moving through even the low points of your fitness journey.

One truism is, the more personal the experience, the more enjoyable it will be. In *Jillian Michaels Fitness Ultimatum 2010,* you have a great deal of control over your workouts, which consist of a series of exercises, in-game background locations, and music. Simply put, if you don't like something, make a change.

In this chapter, you find out about custom and preset Circuit Training as well as custom and preset Resolutions. As you can see, you have many quick-start or personal options to choose from and configure. Get started by taking a look at Circuit Training.

Examining Circuit Training

Circuit Training is accessed from the Workout Area from the Island Hub main menu. Train by using either one of Jillian's included circuits, or one you've set up and saved for yourself by selecting the exercises and the number of repetitions — refer to Chapter 11 for an overview of the available exercises — if you want to include them in your circuit. Figure 12-1 shows the default Circuit Training menu screen, with the five predefined Jillian's Circuits and five empty My Circuits slots that allow you to define and save your own workout routines.

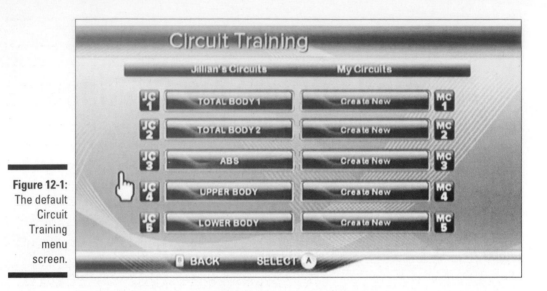

A circuit can have up to nine different exercise combinations from either one or both of the Wii Remote and Wii Balance Board categories as well as one warm-up and one cool-down exercise (see Chapter 1 for more on warming up and cooling down), both of which are required. Finally, a circuit consists of a location and music, both of which are definable on a per-exercise basis.

You can press + on your Wii Remote at any time during an exercise in a circuit to bring up the Pause menu, where you have the choice of continuing, skipping the exercise, or quitting the circuit entirely.

Jillian's Circuits

Jillian's Circuits consist of five targeted workouts: Total Body 1 (Table 12-1), Total Body 2 (Table 12-2), Abs (Table 12-3), Upper Body (Table 12-4), and Lower Body (Table 12-5). The location for every exercise is random, except for Running, which always takes place on the Beach Landing. The music is random for every exercise. The tables below indicate which exercises encompass Jillian's Circuits. After selecting a circuit, such as Total Body 1, shown in Figure 12-2, you are given the opportunity to review but not modify what the workout consists of. Select Start Workout to begin. To exit, press the B button on your Wii Remote.

Table 12-1	Total Body 1 Circuit (JC1)	
Slot	*Exercise*	*Reps/Laps*
0	Running (Warm Up)	5
1	Push-Up	5
2	Lunge Kick	10
3	Push-Up	5
4	Lunge Kick	10
5	Back Kick	10
6	Bicycle	25
7	Crunch	20
8	Swing Kick	10
9	Pelvic Thrust	5
10	Lunge Stretch (Cool Down)	1

Table 12-2	Total Body 2 Circuit (JC2)	
Slot	*Exercise*	*Reps/Laps*
0	Running (Warm Up)	5
1	Water Pump	40
2	Push-Up	15
3	Crunch	20
4	Jumping Jack	30
5	Side Lunge	30
6	Swing Kick	20
7	Oblique	60
8	Bicycle	99
9	Boat Pose	10
10	Lunge Stretch (Cool Down)	1

Table 12-3	Abs (JC3)	
Slot	*Exercise*	*Reps/Laps*
0	Running (Warm Up)	5
1	Jumping Jacks	90
2	Hip Twist	21
3	Bicycle	50
4	Sledge Swing	20
5	Oblique	60
6	Jumping Jack	60
7	Crunch	60
8	Push-Up	15
9	Boat Pose	10
10	Lunge Stretch (Cool Down)	1

Table 12-4	Upper Body (JC4)	
Slot	*Exercise*	*Reps/Laps*
0	Running (Warm Up)	5
1	Push-Up	25
2	Back Kick	20
3	Sledge Swing	20
4	Water Pump	20
5	Running	5
6	Push-Up	25
7	Back Kick	20
8	Sledge Swing	40
9	Boat Pose	20
10	Knees to Chest (Cool Down)	1

Table 12-5	Lower Body (JC5)	
Slot	*Exercise*	*Reps/Laps*
0	Running (Warm Up)	5
1	Lunge Kick	30
2	Swing Kick	30
3	Squat Jacks	30
4	Swing Kick	30
5	Lunge Kick	30
6	Side Lunge	30
7	Jumping Jack	30
8	Side Lunge	30
9	Jumping Jack	30
10	Lunge Stretch (Cool Down)	1

My Circuits

To create your own workout routine, select an empty slot by clicking Create New or, if all of the slots are filled, select an existing circuit to modify. When creating a new circuit, the My Circuit Training screen appears, as shown in Figure 12-2.

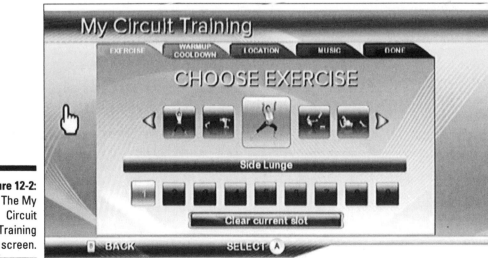

Figure 12-2:
The My Circuit Training screen.

On the Exercise tab, you have a choice of all available exercises (refer to Chapter 11 for an overview of the exercises). Scroll through the choices with either the left or right blue arrow. You can then add any exercise that is in the center of the list by hovering over it with your pointer and pressing A. You are asked to enter the number of repetitions you want to perform on the Reps screen. One such screen, for the Side Lunge, is shown in Figure 12-3. Your rep range is constrained by your choice of Easy, Medium, or Hard, and you can raise or lower your rep range within those limits by clicking on the up and down blue arrows, respectively, or by similarly pressing up and down on your Wii Remote's D-pad. When you're satisfied with your choice, select Done to move on.

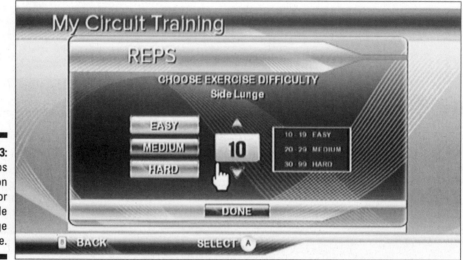

Figure 12-3:
A Reps selection screen for the Side Lunge exercise.

If you want to remove an exercise from one of the nine slots, click the slot in question. After it starts flashing, select Clear current slot to remove it.

If you don't yet have a Balance Board, you may want to design a circuit of only Wii Remote exercises. Of course, not having a Balance Board shouldn't stop you from doing those movements anyway for variety.

Unlike Jillian's Circuits, you don't have to fill all nine slots with exercises. In fact — particularly in the beginning — we recommend that you don't fill all the slots and always pick the lowest possible number of repetitions until you get a feel for what works best with your body's own exercise tolerance.

The same tips for creating your own routines that we give in Chapter 9 for *EA Sports Active: Personal Trainer* also apply when designing your own circuit in *Jillian Michaels Fitness Ultimatum 2010.* Try to design intense workouts that last less than 60 minutes and where you have a clear idea of what body parts you're targeting (see Chapter 11 for what each of the Jillian Michaels exercises target). Rather than detrimentally breaking your body down, getting sufficient rest between workouts and between working the same body parts is key to getting stronger and healthier.

You may just want to mimic Jillian's Circuits based on the tables provided earlier if for nothing else than being able to set your own locations and music.

After you're satisfied with your exercise selections, click on the Warmup Cooldown tab. Your one warm-up choice is Running, though you're able to select your lap range by clicking on the icon and going to the Laps screen. You have a choice of two cool-down exercises, Knees to Chest and the Lunge Stretch, each of which also has its own adjustable rep range. When satisfied, move on to the Location tab.

The Location tab allows you to choose the background Jillian's avatar works out with you in. You can choose a different location for each slot you have an exercise in. When satisfied, move on to the Music tab.

The Music tab works just like the Location tab — one music selection per exercise in a slot. You can preview one of the 20 tracks by clicking the Music Preview bar, which also can be toggled off. Once finished, move on to the last tab, Done.

The Done tab is your last stop in the creation process. You have a chance to view the configuration of each slot with an exercise. Simply click the slot to see the summary of the Exercise, Reps, Location, and Music. If you want to make a change to any of the slots, go back to the appropriate tab and make your change; otherwise, click Save Changes. Input the name you want and then click Enter to save your circuit. This returns you to the Circuit Training screen, where you can then click on your newly created circuit and choose Start Workout to begin working out.

Establishing Resolutions

Resolutions is accessed from the Workout Area from the Island Hub main menu. Here you can set up and edit your Resolutions Calendar or view Jillian's premade resolutions. To ensure consistency in your training, you cannot modify a Resolution after you have saved it. You can only delete the Resolution and start a new one.

When selecting Resolutions, you are presented with an option to continue with the Tutorial On or the Tutorial Off, with the only difference being additional descriptive text at each stage of the process when the tutorial is set to On. Selecting either option brings you to the My Resolution screen, which gives you the option of Create New or Jillian's Pre-Made.

As with the rest of the games mentioned in this book, it is critical to *Jillian Michaels Fitness Ultimatum 2010* that your Wii's date and time are accurate. Please refer to your Wii operations manual that came with your console or, for additional detail, *Wii For Dummies by Kyle Orland* (Wiley Publishing), if you need help setting the date and time.

Create New

Selecting Create New has you start by setting your weekly workout schedule. You are given a seven-day view to work with, which allows you to select up to four different single exercises or circuits for each day of the week. To create a new Resolution, follow these steps:

1. **Scroll over the day of the week you want and press the A button.**

2. **Select the exercises you want to perform on the day by scrolling over a slot and pressing the A button.**

   You have up to four slots you can fill with any combination of single exercises or circuits.

3. **Select Circuit Training or Single Exercise.**

   After you have made your selection, if you want to add additional exercises or a circuit in one of the other available slots, do so now.

4. **When you are satisfied with your day's activities, click the Done button.**

   You can now schedule activities for other days of the week. When you are done with your weekly schedule, click the Start Date button to select the start date on the calendar. After your start date is selected and you click the Accept button, select your end date.

5. **Click the End Date button.**

   A Resolution can be as short as two days or as long as six months.

6. **Enter your end date and click the Accept button.**

7. **If you want to modify any of the information you entered, do so now; otherwise, select Save and Continue and name your Resolution.**

You cannot modify a Resolution after it has been created; you can only delete it. After a Resolution workout is scheduled, you only have the 24-hour calendar day to complete it or it is considered missed.

When you return to the Resolutions screen, you are brought directly to the calendar for your current Resolution, where you can see your latest information or begin a workout. If you have a resolution waiting, as shown in Figure 12-4, you are prompted to Attempt it or simply choose Later if you aren't quite ready for your workout.

Figure 12-4:
A Resolution
Calendar
screen,
showing a
prompt for
a resolution
waiting to be
attempted.

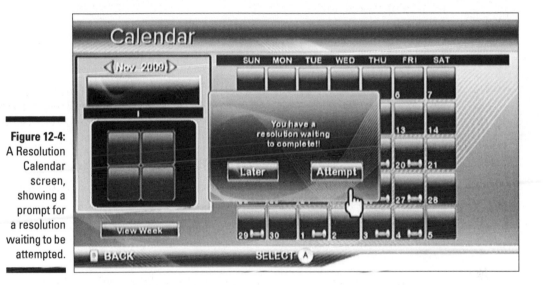

Jillian's Pre-Made

Selecting Jillian's Pre-Made resolutions presents you with four options: Arms, Back, and Chest, which takes place over a period of one month; Back 2 Basics, which takes place over two months; Total Body Workout, which takes place over three months; and Ultimate 6, which takes place over the maximum six-month schedule. Naturally, Arms, Back, and Chest rates the easiest, while Ultimate 6 rates the hardest, so choose a Resolution based on your experience level.

These premade resolutions also provide great guidance for creating your own schedule, so don't be afraid to tackle the game's customization features after you go through one or two of these. Remember, although resolutions shouldn't be made to be broken, they can easily be deleted if you don't like how they're designed — and you can try, try again!

Part IV
The Part of Tens

The 5th Wave   By Rich Tennant

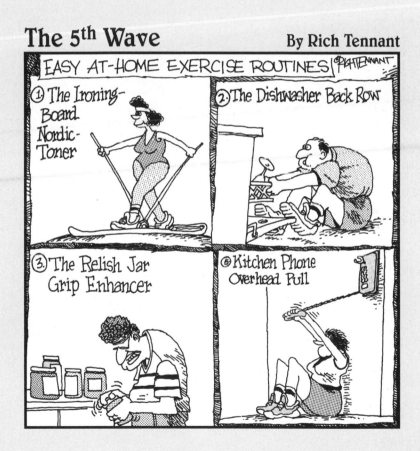

In this part . . .

This part brings your Wii fitness journey to a fitting conclusion by helping to both enhance your experience and also keep it going indefinitely. You learn about the Wii fitness accessories that can make both your general Nintendo Wii play more enjoyable, as well as enhance your Wii fitness workouts. Finally, you find out about many of the ever expanding number of other available Wii fitness games. Remember, if you keep on following the advice in this book, you'll ensure that it's only the games doing the expanding and not you!

Chapter 13

Ten Best Wii Fitness Accessories

. . . .

*T*hroughout this book, we show you how to maximize your Wii fitness experience. Now, you can accessorize it. One of the key tips to sticking with any exercise regime is keeping the experience fresh and fun to ensure that both your mind and body remain in the game.

Of course, some of these accessories are of the more practical variety, such as the rechargeable battery packs, while others, like the aerobics step risers, specifically enhance the difficulty level and effectiveness of games that use the Balance Board. Regardless of whether you implement one or all of these accessories now or in the future, we are sure you'll agree that having so many options is nice.

Getting Down

Although the primary functionality of *Wii Fit Plus* is centered around the use of the Balance Board, which many other Wii fitness titles also support, you're just as likely to be off the board as you are on it. For this reason, making your off-board experience — particularly floor work — as comfortable as possible is important. Exercise mats can help. Even a lightly padded mat can make working out on the floor a more pleasant experience, all while providing additional traction.

Many types of mats, including sticky, extra-thick, phthalate- and latex-free, eco-friendly, and printed are available. You have numerous choices when you're looking for a mat that is best suited to your specific needs. However, the main characteristics you want to look for in a mat are padding and traction, because those two areas of functionality tend to be the most critical, particularly when performing yoga exercises. The following list covers the categories of mat options.

✔ **Sticky:** Most good mats have some type of non-slip gripping surface, either on one or both sides. Generally speaking, these mats provide a fair amount of traction on any surface, even rugs, which is important when you're trying to hold a specific position. Keep in mind that cheaper mats often have slicker surfaces.

✔ **Extra-thick:** The thicker the mat, the more cushioning is provided, something you'll appreciate when your knees are digging into the ground. Typical mat thickness starts at ⅛ inch, while thicker mats start at ¼ inch and can go to ½ inch or higher. Of course one downside to a thicker mat — particularly ones designed for pilates — is that you start to lose feel for the floor, a critical component of the types of yoga exercises you perform in *Wii Fit Plus,* for example. More expensive mats often contain air pockets rather than foam to provide better and longer-lasting cushioning.

✔ **Phthalate-and latex-free:** Phthalates are substances added to plastics to increase their flexibility, transparency, durability, and longevity. Because phthalates are being phased out in the United States over health concerns, it's best to look for mats that are already free of such substances. Latex, on the other hand, is a natural or synthetic substance used to make rubber that is considered safe unless you have a specific allergy, in which case it also becomes a material to avoid when selecting a mat.

✔ **Eco-friendly:** Being in tune with your body often translates into being more in tune with the world around you, so a mat made from Earth-friendly recycled material may be a good choice for you. Although these types of mats tend to cost more, they are typically fully biodegradable and latex-free.

✔ **Printed:** Most exercise mats feature textured surfaces in single, solid colors, but some, particularly premium mats, can feature elaborate designs or patterns. If you want something more decorative or provocative while you work out, keep an eye out for a design that personally appeals to you. Unfortunately, even if you find an appealing design, it may not have one of the other properties — such as being eco-friendly or extra-thick — that you're looking for, so it's best in this case to choose function over form, if you're forced to choose.

Exercise mats are available from a wide variety of retailers, with some of the more specialized mats typically available only from yoga or pilates suppliers. Prices generally start around $10, with prices exceeding $100 for the fanciest mats. Somewhere under $40 tends to be the sweet spot for both price and performance.

Using Eco- and Econo-Friendly Power

The wireless nature of the Balance Board comes with a price — the eventual conspicuous consumption of batteries. As mentioned in Chapter 1, the Balance Board requires four AA batteries, which is the equivalent power of two Wii Remotes. The solution to this is to go with a rechargeable battery option, either rechargeable batteries or a special rechargeable battery pack.

Although rechargeable batteries have a higher initial cost, they can be recharged many times during their service life — from approximately 100 to more than 1,000 charge cycles depending upon type and brand. Use of rechargeables can greatly reduce the amount of toxic materials sent to landfills compared with the equivalent number of disposable batteries that would be required for the same usage period. Let's take a look at some of the rechargeable battery options for the Balance Board:

- ✓ **Standard NiMH rechargeable batteries** cost approximately $10 to $20 for four and require a charger ($15 and up), but are sometimes available in a combination package at a reduced cost ($15 and up). Keep an eye out for rechargeable batteries that promise more than 1,000 recharges for maximum value. Keeping extra rechargeable batteries on hand always gives you access to power even while your other batteries are charging and also makes a great addition to your Wii Remotes.

- ✓ **The CTA Digital WI-BBP Battery Pack** ($19.99) is a single unit that plugs into the Balance Board's battery compartment. The CTA Digital battery pack is charged by using the included USB cable from any powered USB port, such as one on your Wii console. The unit can be charged while the Balance Board is being used.

- ✓ **The Nyko Wii Fit Energy Pak** ($29.99) is a single unit much like CTA's offering, but instead of charging via USB, it charges via a regular AC power outlet for quicker recharges.

Of course, besides generally maxing out at approximately half the rated 60-hour battery life of disposables between every charge, the major trade-off to using some type of rechargeable solution is that you need to remember to keep it charged!

Rechargeable battery solutions aren't just for the Balance Board, either. A plethora of rechargeable options is available for your Wii Remote as well, from standard batteries that start around $10 for a pack of four without a charger or around $20 with one, to elaborate docking stations such as the Intec Nintendo Wii Charger Dock with four Battery Packs, which starts around $30. With the right combination of products, you can sever your Wii's dependence on disposable batteries forever.

Keeping It Covered

Whether you use it with or without the Wii MotionPlus accessory, your Wii Remote should always be used with the Wii Remote Jacket for maximum safety. Although the Balance Board is designed to be used without a cover, adding a silicone, rubber, or plastic sleeve can add a touch of style, reduce wear and tear on both you and the board, and provide extra traction. Of course, removable covers are also much easier to clean and all exercisers can have their own board covers for optimal hygiene.

Most covers are available in a variety of colors, as well as clear, and some even glow in the dark. The typically soft materials help to absorb impacts better than just the board alone, which is particularly nice on your feet during long step aerobics sessions. Covers are available from a variety of manufacturers, including CTA Digital, GamerGearOnline.com, Talismoon, WC, and YoungMicro. Major differences between brands include color, texture, and price.

Getting a Grip

As mentioned in Chapter 1, the Balance Board is best used with bare feet, even though using socks is more hygienic. Although the board does provide traction, the risk of slipping in regular socks is too great. If you are ashamed of your feet, they tend to get cold, or they become sweaty and slippery, consider investing in a pair of non-slip socks, such as the ones from CTA Digital, DreamGear, or Hyperkin. Of course, there is a downside to even non-slip socks, as they can inhibit achieving optimal balance by preventing your toes from separating. However, there is a solution: toe socks, which are worn by the authors in this book's photos.

Form fitting yoga or pilates toe socks not only provide a non-slip surface, but also allow a more complete range of motion. By allowing the toes to wiggle freely, the muscles in the foot can also become more flexible and stronger. Some toe socks even feature a horizontal stripe to help with alignment, which is particularly useful for certain *Wii Fit Plus* exercises. Toe socks are also available in half-toe varieties, where everything but your toes is covered. Brands include Acacia, Stick-E, ToeSox, and Yoga Paws.

With your feet receiving so much attention, are your hands feeling left out? If you find that even with the Wii Remote's strap and jacket you're still a sweaty butterfingers, consider non-slip gloves or grips, which, like non-slip socks, are also great for getting extra traction on floor exercises. Non-slip grips are available in full glove, fingerless, or palm-only varieties, and are available from manufacturers such as Stick-E, Sun Salutations, and Yoga Paws. Prices start around $15 per pair.

Creating Tension

EA Sports Active: Personal Trainer is centered around the use of its included Resistance Band. Although the EA Sports Active: Accessory Pack, discussed in Chapter 7, contains a second Resistance Band, it also contains a second Leg Strap, which makes it redundant and expensive for anything other than as a full replacement set or as a set for a second player. If you're looking for just a Resistance Band replacement, either because yours is broken and beyond the 90-day warranty period or you want something that offers more resistance, you need to look outside of the EA offerings. Luckily, resistance bands are a common exercise accessory, particularly for pilates enthusiasts, and a range of options is widely available.

You can find two basic types of resistance bands: the flat, ribbon style, such as the type that comes with *EA Sports Active: Personal Trainer,* and a shape more like thin rubber tubing. Other than personal preference, you won't find major differences between the two types. Some, like Aylio's Resistance Bands Exercise Training Set, include a range of bands that offer varying levels of resistance and a strap-style handle similar to the EA default option, which makes holding the Wii Remote easier. There are also other, lower-cost options, such as the Dyna-Band brand resistance bands that come in different resistance levels and offer the same style of band that EA does, even fitting into the same black straps.

Although you get the most use out of resistance bands in *EA Sports Active: Personal Trainer* because it was explicitly designed around their use, you can easily incorporate them into most other Wii fitness software when you want a different type of challenge.

Moving on Up

If you find that *Wii Fit Plus*'s step aerobics exercises, discussed in Chapter 5 — or any of the other programs' exercises that involve stepping up onto the Balance Board — have become too easy, there is a solution for you. Adding a simple riser to your Balance Board allows you to raise the board to a height of four inches, which is standard in most step aerobics classes. Although not its intended purpose, in a pinch, these risers can also provide a higher and more stable platform on thicker rugs than the Wii Balance Board Foot Extensions.

Widely available aerobics step risers for the Balance Board include the CTA Digital 3-inch Aerobics Step Platform for Wii Fit, Everlast 3-inch Aerobic Step, and ZooZen Riiser Wii Fit Balance Board Aerobic Step.

Of Brassards and Remotes

If you use any of the myriad Wii fitness programs for any stretch of time, you may notice one major annoyance over all others — having nowhere to put your Wii Remote while performing the various exercises. Because, at minimum, the Wii Remote is required for menu navigation, there's really no way around its constant use. One clever solution to the issue of picking up and putting down your Wii Remote or holding it in your hand most of the time is an idea borrowed from those who work out with MP3 players such as Apple's iPod — arm bands.

As of this writing, the most widely available arm band is the Wiitality Armband, which can fit over your biceps or wrist, the latter of which is the best location for programs such as *EA Sports Active: Personal Trainer*. This neoprene band holds your Wii Remote while you exercise, and leaves the buttons on the top of the remote fully accessible.

Breaking Free

Because both your Wii Remote and Balance Board are such wonders of wireless technology, it's something of a disappointment when you get to an activity like *Wii Fit Plus*'s Rhythm Boxing, described in Chapter 5, and discover you need to attach the Nunchuk to your remote with a cable. Luckily, it's easy to liberate your Nunchuk from its Wii Remote bondage. The following list describes a few of the available options to allow you to play more footloose and fancy free. Try these options:

- **Nyko Cord-Free for Wii Nunchuk** converts your existing wired Nunchuk into a wireless peripheral by placing it into a self-standing sleeve that also acts as storage. This Nyko device runs on two AAA batteries, promising up to 60 hours of run-time.

- **Nyko Wireless Kama** is a stand-alone Nunchuk-compatible device that runs on two AAA batteries for up to 30 hours of run-time.

- **Icon Wireless Playchuk Pro** is a stand-alone, rechargeable Nunchuk-compatible device with a built-in battery. Any powered USB port — such as the one on your Wii console — charges the device via the included cable. An LED charge indicator shows when the battery is charging.

- **Intec Wireless Nunchuk** is another stand-alone, rechargeable Nunchuk-compatible device with a built-in battery, but features a more traditional design, similar to Nintendo's Nunchuk.

Wireless Nunchuk solutions are available from most retailers that carry Nintendo Wii products.

All of the presently available wireless Nunchuk solutions, regardless of whether they adapt an existing wired controller or are stand-alone devices, require that a small receiver be plugged into the bottom of your Wii Remote. Keep in mind that these receivers may or may not be compatible with your current Wii Remote Jacket or anything else you might place your Wii Remote into, such as the weights described in the next section. The Leg Strap for *EA Sports Active: Personal Trainer* may also have issues with non-standard Nunchuk shapes, so it's important to do research before deciding on which wireless solution is right for you.

Wireless products that use a 2.4 GHz wireless frequency may be prone to interference from other devices, such as cordless phones or microwave ovens.

Heavy Handed

Earlier in this chapter, we mention that one way to up your workout intensity with the Balance Board is to use an aerobics step riser. Although this is a great solution for working your lower body and overall cardiorespiratory system, an excellent alternative or adjunct to this is to put more focus on your upper body by turning your Wii Remote and Nunchuk into dumbbells. There are presently two solutions, each of which maintains full controller functionality while in use:

- ✔ **Power Play Corporation RiiFlex** dumbbell pair comes in both 2-lb. (green) and 4-lb. (blue) options, with one dumbbell holding Nintendo's standard Wii Remote, without a Wii Remote Jacket, and the other dumbbell holding Nintendo's standard Nunchuk.

- ✔ **Everlast 2lb Dumbbells** provide a lower cost alternative to the RiiFlex, but currently come in only one size and feature more traditional styling

Even though programs such as *Wii Fit Plus* have you to use the Nunchuk for only a few activities, such as Rhythm Parade discussed in Chapter 6, and *EA Sports Active: Personal Trainer* often has you place the Nunchuk in the Leg Strap, to maximize the effectiveness of these weights, try to hold both dumbbells whenever possible. One nice feature about the added weight to your Wii Remote and Nunchuk is that you can make use of them even outside of the Wii fitness programs for just about any other Wii-related activities.

Safety and form are always your two top priorities. If you find you're getting tired or the weights become too heavy to move correctly, immediately switch to using the Wii Remote and Nunchuk normally, or simply take a breather.

Of course, there are many other options for adding weight to your Wii fitness regimen, including wrist and ankle weights and weight vests. Naturally, if you use any of these heavy accessories, be sure to weigh yourself on the Balance Board before using them, and make sure that your combined weight does not exceed the board's 330-lb. limit.

Stepping Out

Studies have shown that pedometers not only encourage users to walk more, but also to move more. For some, a pedometer might reinforce behavior change; for others, it may simply act as a wearable reminder to stick with the healthier lifestyle that began with *Wii Fitness For Dummies*. If you can instantly check how you're progressing based on data from even a tiny device like a pedometer, the immediate satisfaction you receive can pay huge dividends, and *Wii Fit Plus* allows you to log your steps. Turn to Chapter 2 for more on this.

Although most pedometers count each step a person takes by detecting the hip motion, some pedometers can be tuned to detect aerobics steps or other types of motion, usually by adjusting the step-length setting. These pedometers can be used even when engaging in a Wii fitness activity, allowing you to log every step that you take. What follows are descriptions of a few of the more interesting low-cost pedometers:

- **Omron HJ-112 Pedometer:** The HJ-112 allows for flexibility in wearing or carrying the device, a plus when doing activities other than walking. The pedometer counts steps — including aerobics steps — and calculates distance and calories burned. The device has a seven-day memory.

- **Yamax Digiwalker CW-701 Pedometer:** The CW-701, known for its ruggedness and step counting accuracy, displays distance, calories burned, and both actual and activity time. The pedometer has a seven-day daily memory and keeps two weeks' worth of totals. The device has a two-line display.

- **Omron HJ-720ITC Pedometer:** The HJ-720ITC tracks the same type of data as the other two devices, but also has an upload feature that allows you to keep track of your data, set goals, and see your progress in a more visual manner via graphs and charts on your personal computer.

Prices for these pedometers start at around $25, and they are available from a variety of retailers.

You often hear about a daily target of 10,000 steps when using a pedometer. This was proposed as a standard because it's the approximate number of steps an average adult human would take if he or she walked at a brisk pace for 30 minutes. As always, because there is no universal gauge for an individual's fitness requirements, adjust this target up or down depending upon your own needs for a given day, week, or circumstance.

Chapter 14

Ten Other Wii Fitness Workout Programs

● ●

Although this book covers three of the most popular Wii fitness titles in *Wii Fit Plus, EA Sports Active: Personal Trainer,* and *Jillian Michaels Fitness Ultimatum 2010,* these are by no means your only options. Besides the original *Wii Fit* and *Jillian Michaels Fitness Ultimatum 2009,* and the expansion pack for *EA Sports Active: Personal Trainer, EA Sports Active: More Workouts,* there are plenty of other ways to satisfy your Wii fitness needs.

Some of these programs function more like interactive workout DVDs, while others are considerably more advanced and come with their own accessories.

Active Life

Namco Bandai's Active Life games, which consist of 2008's *Active Life: Outdoor Challenge* and 2009's *Active Life: Extreme Challenge,* each come with something called the Active Life mat. In conjunction with the Wii Remote, the large mat allows one or two players to control the onscreen action with their hands and feet. Unlike the rigid Balance Board, the flexible Active Life mat is more like the popular dance pad controllers that support running and jumping. Unlike dance pads, which are typically intended for one person, the Active Life mat supports up to two players at once. Although the Active Life games are targeted primarily to children, the activities can be enjoyed by the entire family.

The Active Life games feature a training mode for different body parts, but they're less about traditional workouts and more about having what we call *active fun.*

Daisy Fuentes Pilates

Pilates has many similarities to yoga in form and function, but it puts more emphasis on deep breathing and the flow, or transition, between each new movement or exercise. Although a popular exercise method, no Wii fitness title specifically addressed the discipline until Sega's *Daisy Fuentes Pilates* in 2009. *Daisy Fuentes Pilates* is one of several celebrity-endorsed fitness titles available for the Wii and makes use of the Wii Remote and, optionally, the Balance Board, though the latter is required to be scored on some of the ten different exercises. Designed exclusively for a single player, *Daisy Fuentes Pilates* offers varying difficulty levels, preset routines, and customizable workouts.

DanceDanceRevolution

Konami's *DanceDanceRevolution* series began life in 1998 as a breakthrough arcade dancing game, but quickly made its way home. The only major difference between the arcade machines and the home conversions is that instead of a metal dance pad, home users typically use flexible dance pads that often come packaged with the games, though a wide variety are also available for purchase separately.

The Wii's *DanceDanceRevolution* titles consist of *Hottest Party* (2007), *Hottest Party 2* (2008), *Disney Grooves* (2009), and *Hottest Party 3* (2009). While primarily fun dancing games where the goal is to step on the appropriate spot on the dance pad when prompted, dance games can really test your cardiovascular endurance when playing the higher levels and even feature workout modes.

Gold's Gym Cardio Workout

Ubisoft's *Gold's Gym Cardio Workout* title from 2009 takes more than a little inspiration from the original *Wii Fit* by also offering a virtual personal training experience, but with a primary focus on cardiovascular exercises, particularly as they relate to how a boxer might train. The control options are varied and include one Wii Remote and the Nunchuk, or two Wii Remotes, with additional support for the Balance Board.

Exercises feature a range of activities, including cardio boxing, running, sit-ups, squats, and log cutting. The program tracks your progress and the difficulty level evolves accordingly.

My Fitness Coach

Ubisoft's *My Fitness Coach,* released in 2008, is perhaps the most hardcore of all Wii fitness programs, but also makes the least use of the platform's features. Instead of incorporating the Wii Remote and Nunchuk — let alone the

Balance Board — *My Fitness Coach* instead asks what exercise equipment you have available. These might include items such as a heart monitor, stability ball, or free weights, with *My Fitness Coach* then customizing your routine from a list of almost 500 unique exercises. The program also guides you in taking various body part measurements, which are used in determining your fitness levels and helps to further customize your workouts to target problem areas.

Because *My Fitness Coach* does not rely on specific Wii accessories, it is able to feature a Group Exercise mode that supports up to four players. Of course, whether four people can work out comfortably in front of your TV is entirely dependent on how much space you have available.

The Biggest Loser

The third Wii fitness title to feature Jillian Michaels, THQ's *The Biggest Loser,* released in 2009, is of course based on the hit NBC television series. *The Biggest Loser* makes good use of the familiar license, allowing you to compete with contestants from past seasons in 4-, 8-, or 12-week programs, or with another player in weekly challenges. The game features more than 88 exercises that focus on upper and lower body, core, cardio, and yoga, with 66 of them able to incorporate the Balance Board.

Besides the typical workout customization and calendar features often found in these types of programs, *The Biggest Loser* also helps you count calories and offers a selection of 50 healthy recipes from one of the brand's cookbooks.

Walk It Out

Walk It Out is a 2009 release from Konami, so it's no surprise that besides supporting the Wii Remote, Nunchuk, and Balance Board, it also supports dance pads. The easiest way to picture *Walk It Out* is as a lower intensity version of the *DanceDanceRevolution* games, where timing is still important, but how quickly you react isn't. Although it's arguable how much exercise benefit there is to simply walking, *Walk It Out* is designed to ratchet up the intensity, which is a key to providing better results.

Walk It Out also jazzes up the experience by featuring more than 100 songs and an interesting game world, where the more you step, the more the environment opens up, with a large list of locations to explore and goodies to uncover. If you're looking for a Wii fitness program with less intensity, but one that still provides some nice cardiovascular benefits and multiplayer support, *Walk It Out* is worth checking out.

Wii Sports

Although not specifically designed around fitness, Nintendo's Wii pack-in game, *Wii Sports* (2006), and it successor, *Wii Sports Resort* (2009), which comes packaged with the Wii MotionPlus controller add-on, will definitely get you moving. Although it serves as a low-impact alternative to specific Wii fitness programs, many of the same types of activities, like boxing and tennis, are available, just in a different context.

On days you may not wish to do a traditional workout or are unable to make it outdoors to do something, playing either of the Wii Sports games is a fine alternative to simply passively sitting in front of the TV.

Yoga

Much like *Daisy Fuentes Pilates,* Dreamcatcher Interactive's *Yoga,* released in 2009, focuses on one specific discipline and runs with it. *Yoga,* more so than Nintendo's *Wii Fit* series, places serious focus on the Zen-like aspects of the practice, showcasing real-life guru Anja Rubik along with an animated avatar. Besides the expected variety of yoga exercises, *Yoga* also provides the philosophical basis behind the practice, encouraging overall well-being.

As a slower, more relaxing approach to yoga, *Yoga* provides a logical next step for those intrigued by what was provided in the *Wii Fit* games. Whether a concession to the more personal, spiritual nature of the game, or more likely due to it requiring the Balance Board, *Yoga* is a strictly single-player experience.

Your Shape

Ubisoft's *Your Shape* (2009) takes a fresh technological approach to fitness by including a camera that scans and projects your image onto your TV in real time next to your virtual workout buddy and guide, celebrity Jenny McCarthy. As such, this single-player game is performed entirely controller-free since your movements are tracked solely with the camera, allowing *Your Shape* to actively correct your form.

Although the camera can be adversely affected by factors in your room, such as poor lighting or a busy background, when you combine its personalization options with close to 500 exercises, *Your Shape* still makes a strong case for inclusion in your Wii fitness arsenal.

Index

Have fun while getting fit! Here's how to get the most from your Wii Fitness system

It's a perfect fit — Wii gaming fun designed to improve your overall health and fitness! The advice of these two personal trainers makes it even better. You'll learn to use *Wii Fit Plus, EA Sports Active: Personal Trainer,* and *Jillian Michaels Fitness Ultimatum 2010*. Find out how to create your own individualized workout and watch yourself improve!

- *What's all this stuff?* — **set up Wii Fit™ Plus, EA Sports™ Active: Personal Trainer, and Jillian Michaels Fitness Ultimatum 2010**

- *The right way* — **learn the safest and most effective way to perform dozens of exercises**

- *Spice it up* — **explore different types of exercises to keep your routine fresh**

- *Take a deep breath* — **improve health benefits by learning optimal breathing techniques**

- *Have a heart* — **strengthen your heart and lungs while enjoying the challenge of sports**

- *A delicate balance* — **identify routines that improve your balance while strengthening different muscle groups**

- *All season sports* — **experience volleyball, baseball, boxing, tennis, inline skating, and basketball right in your living room**

- *Keep it interesting* — **vary your workout by moving among the featured games**

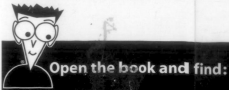

Open the book and find:

- Ways to vary your routine
- How to set up your Fitness Profile
- Tips for staying motivated
- The power of yoga and strength training
- What to consider when setting fitness goals
- Warm-up and cool-down routines
- How to build your own workout
- Ten cool Wii Fitness accessories
- Ten other Wii Fitness games to expand your virtual gym

Go to Dummies.com®
for videos, step-by-step examples, how-to articles, or to shop!

For Dummies®
A Branded Imprint of
⊕WILEY

$21.99 US / $25.99 CN / £16.99 UK

ISBN 978-0-470-52158-8

52199

9 780470 521588

Christina T. Loguidice is Editor of *Oncology Net Guide* and *OncNurse* and holds a Black Belt in Tae Kwon Do. **Bill Loguidice** is cofounder and Managing Director for the online publication *Armchair Arcade* (www.armchairarcade.com). Both are American Fitness Training of Athletics (AFTA) Certified Personal Trainers.